D0886642

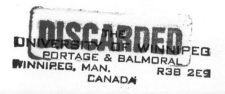

DISCARDED

THE
UNIVERSITY OF WINNIPEG
PORTAGE & BALMORAL
WINNIPEG, MAN.   R3B 2E9
CANADA

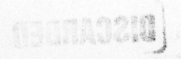
DISCARDED

Psychiatry and Psychology in the USSR

RC
451
·R9P79

Psychiatry and Psychology in the USSR

Edited by
Samuel A. Corson
The Ohio State University, Columbus

Associate editor
Elizabeth O'Leary Corson
The Ohio State University, Columbus

PLENUM PRESS · NEW YORK AND LONDON

Library of Congress Cataloging in Publication Data

Main entry under title:

Psychiatry and psychology in the USSR.

"Proceedings of a symposium convened at the Ohio State University, Columbus, Ohio, April 25, 1975 under the auspices of the Ohio State University Center for Slavic and Eastern European Studies and the Departments of Psychiatry and Psychology."
Includes index.
1. Psychiatry—Russia—Congresses, 2. Psychology—Russia—Congresses.
I. Corson, Samuel Abraham, 1909-   II. Corson, Elizabeth O'Leary.
III. Ohio. State University, Columbus. Center for Slavic and Eastern European Studies. IV. Ohio. State University, Columbus. Dept. of Psychiatry. V. Ohio. State University, Columbus. Dept. of Psychology.
[DNLM: 1. Psychiatry—U. S. S. R.—Congresses. 2. Psychology—U.S.S.R.—Congresses. WM100 P98613 1975]
RC451.R9P79   616.8'9'00947   76-47482
ISBN 0-306-30992-0

Proceedings of a symposium convened at the Ohio State University,
Columbus, Ohio, April 25, 1975 under the auspices of the
Ohio State University Center for Slavic and Eastern European Studies
and the Departments of Psychiatry and Psychology

©1976 Plenum Press, New York
A Division of Plenum Publishing Corporation
227 West 17th Street, New York, N.Y. 10011

All rights reserved

No part of this book may be reproduced, stored in a retrieval system, or transmitted, in any form or by any means, electronic, mechanical, photocopying, microfilming, recording, or otherwise, without written permission from the Publisher

Printed in the United States of America

This volume is dedicated to

DR. W. HORSLEY GANTT

A pioneer in the development of
Pavlovian psychobiology
and
biological psychiatry

Acknowledgments

We wish to acknowledge with gratitude our indebtedness to Professor Ian Gregory, Chairman of our Department of Psychiatry, for his encouragement in the organization of this symposium and the preparation and editing of this volume. Professor Leon I. Twarog, Director of the Center for Slavic and East European Studies at our University, was largely responsible for suggesting the idea for this symposium and providing financial resources and the impetus for its implementation.

To Mr. Roland Dartau we are grateful for his careful proofreading and his expert assistance with bibliographic references and indexing, particularly with those items dealing with Russian sources. We thank Mr. Charles G. Brugh for his assistance with the typing of the index.

Preface

This book is aimed at a professional audience of psychiatrists, psychologists, and educators, as well as Slavic studies scholars and teachers and intelligent lay readers.

It would be presumptious to attempt to cover the entire field of Soviet psychiatry and psychology in one modest volume. During the past several decades there has been a remarkable flourishing and diversification of research in psychology and psychiatry in the USSR. What we have attempted to do in this symposium is to present a constructive critical overview of certain limited areas by arranging an interchange of observations and ideas between several American scientists knowledgeable in these fields and a psychologist and psychiatrist who obtained their education and working experience in the USSR. We hope to be able to expand such symposia in the future, so as to cover other important areas of these disciplines.

This monograph presents an eyewitness account of Pavlov by W. Horsley Gantt, one of three surviving students of Pavlov, and, to the best of my knowledge, the only American who actually studied and worked with Pavlov. It is a measure of Dr. Gantt's devotion to the development of scientific psychiatry that he went to the USSR to spend six years in Pavlov's laboratory at a time of extreme economic hardship and political turmoil in that country and in the face of having to master a difficult language. In his presentation, Dr. Gantt also summarizes his own contributions and those of his students to the extension and broadening of Pavlovian methods and concepts and their applications to the development of biological psychiatry.

Philosophical and historical roots of Pavlovian psycho-biology are reviewed by the editors of this volume. Josef Brožek presents an elegant review of historiography of Soviet psychology and of Pavloviana in the USA. Robert M. Krauss, a distinguished social psychologist, presents a

succinct outline of the major categories of Soviet research
in social psychology. He calls attention to the fact that
social psychology in the USSR has a strong theoretical orientation and is directed primarily to field studies rather
than to contrived laboratory experiments so characteristic
of a good deal of social psychology research in the USA.

Elkhonon Goldberg, a student of the outstanding Soviet
neuropsychologist, A. R. Luria, presents a detailed and
scholarly survey of the philosophical background and the
techniques of neuropsychologic and behavioral tests devised
by the Luria school of defectology. This includes descriptions of tests of cognitive defects and motor processes
after brain lesions. Dr. Goldberg also points out the
theoretical underpinning of clinical psychology in the USSR
as contrasted with the empirical applied orientation in
American clinical psychology.

Robert H. Wozniak, an authority in cognitive developmental psychology, contrasts the developmental dialectic
analysis of intelligence in the USSR with the psychometric
"fixed capacity" approach prevailing in the USA. He points
out the similarity of the approach of Soviet psychologists
to that of Piaget.

Jimmie Holland and Isidore Ziferstein, two distinguished
American psychiatrists, present descriptions of their experiences while working as psychiatrists in two of the major
psychiatric clinical centers in the USSR. Dr. Holland spent
a year in 1972-73 at a large psychiatric hospital in Moscow
as a consultant for the National Institute of Mental Health.
Dr. Ziferstein spent 13 months in 1963-64 in the USSR at the
famous Bekhterev Psychoneurological Institute in Leningrad
under a fellowship from the Foundations Fund for Research in
Psychiatry. Dr. Holland's presentation includes a comparison
of Soviet and American modes of medical and psychiatric
education and training and of principles guiding diagnosis
and classification of mental diseases. She points out that,
while a single care system in the USSR permits early detection of mental illness and assurance of follow-up and continuing care, that system has apparently not made provisions
for safeguarding legal rights of the patients.

Dr. Ziferstein presents a vivid description of the
historical and philosophical orientation of Soviet psychiatry
and of daily interactions between the psychiatrist and the
patient. He analyzes the active role assumed by a Soviet

psychiatrist, as contrasted with the traditional nondirective, purely interpretive role of classical psychoanalysis. Dr. Ziferstein also gives a good description of Soviet collective psychotherapy as compared to group therapy practiced in the USA.

Boris Segal, an outstanding Soviet psychiatrist and an authority on alcoholism, recently emigrated to the USA. In his paper on "Drinking Patterns and Alcoholism in Soviet and American Societies," Dr. Segal presents a scholarly, well documented analysis of the interaction of biological, cultural, socio-economic, and political factors involved in alcoholism in the two countries, including a comparison of methods of research, treatment, and prevention.

Finally, Boris Segal presents a balanced, carefully documented critical review of a highly controversial subject, namely the problem of involuntary hospitalization of political dissidents in Soviet psychiatric hospitals. After documenting cases of compulsory psychiatric hospitalization of Soviet dissidents, Segal emphasizes that such politicization of psychiatry is not characteristic of the overwhelming majority of Soviet psychiatrists, whose medical and ethical standards are comparable to those of physicians in Western countries. Moreover, Segal points out that psychiatric incarceration of political dissidents testifies to the relative liberalization of the regime, since these occasional abuses of psychiatry are not to be compared with the Stalinist terror when millions of innocent, even apolitical, people were physically exterminated without any pretense of judicial procedure.

It is well to keep this thought in mind. Deplorable as psychiatric incarceration of political dissidents is, it is certainly not warranted to assume that placement of political dissidents in prisons or labor camps is any more civilized, whether it occurs in the USSR or in any other country, whether it be in Europe, Asia, or the American continent.

In the long run, the elimination of political repression of any kind in any country could probably best be achieved by universal relaxation of international tensions and the elimination of reliance on armaments and escalation of armament races as major expressions of foreign policies of various states, particularly of the so-called great powers.

In the words of the Quaker William Penn,

        Love and persuasion have more force
        Than weapons of war,
        Nor would the worst of men
        Easily be brought to hurt those
        That they really think love them.
        It is that love and patience
        Which must in the end have victory...

Samuel A. Corson
Department of Psychiatry
College of Medicine
The Ohio State University
Columbus, Ohio

Contents

INTRODUCTORY REMARKS

Leon I. Twarog

Center for Slavic and East European Studies

The Ohio State University, Columbus, Ohio

Each spring the Center for Slavic and East European Studies at The Ohio State University sponsors a one-day Symposium on a topical subject which also reflects the special expertise of its faculty. The Center has as its central mission the development of Slavic and East European Studies throughout the State of Ohio at all academic levels, from the secondary school through the graduate school. It coordinates the activities of more than 50 faculty members from 20 departments and 7 colleges on the campus of The Ohio State University, and fosters cooperative ventures among them and faculty from other colleges and universities in Ohio and the nation.

The Annual Symposium provides a fortuitous setting for the generation of new knowledge about the Soviet Union and Eastern Europe and the simultaneous transmission of this knowledge to the broadest possible audience of students, faculty, and the general citizenry. Few universities in this country have on their faculties a specialist in either psychology or psychiatry in the Soviet Union and Eastern Europe, but at The Ohio State University both fields are represented by scholars who have been following developments in their respective areas for several years, and who regularly teach in their areas of specialization as well. Dr. Timothy Brock, Professor of Psychology, regularly teaches a course on Psychology in the USSR; Dr. Samuel Corson, Professor of Psychiatry and Biophysics, has taken time out from his busy schedule in the research laboratory to take students with him on study tours to Eastern Europe and the

USSR, so that students might take advantage of the relations he has built up over the years with the leading research laboratories in Eastern Europe and the Soviet Union.

Professor Brock and Professor Corson were given the task of preparing a program for the Symposium--the fruits of which comprise this volume, the first of its kind to appear in several years.

WELCOME AND INTRODUCTION

Ian Gregory

Department of Psychiatry
The Ohio State University
Columbus, Ohio

On behalf of The Ohio State University Department of
Psychiatry, it is a great pleasure to join with Doctor
Twarog and Doctor Osipow in welcoming our distinguished colleagues on today's program and the audience that has come
to hear and learn.

Abnormal thinking, feeling, and behavior are defined
as such by the society in which the individual lives. Attempts to prevent, modify, or eliminate such abnormality
depend on prevailing social beliefs as well as available
technological resources. All these have changed dramatically
within our own society during my own professional career
(which covers roughly the time span since the end of World
War II).

Differences between psychiatric evaluation and treatment in North America in the late 1940s and in the early
1970s are at least as profound as those likely to be found
between two technologically advanced countries at the present time. Ours is a complex and pluralistic society, which
has fostered the simultaneous development of different approaches to the same problem. We have often concluded that
there is more than one way to skin a cat and more than one
entrance to the city of truth.

Moreover, it is recognized that major differences
exist between psychiatry and psychology in English-speaking
countries. The same disorder may be labeled or diagnosed dif-
ferently in the United States and the United Kingdom, may be

3

attributed to different causal factors, and treated by different approaches.

It would be surprising indeed if theoretical and pragmatic differences, at least as obvious as these, did not exist between psychiatry as practiced in the United States and in the Soviet Union. However, there may also be substantial and even surprising similarities.

We are here today to learn what we may from our distinguished speakers, and I would urge that we make every effort to shed our prejudices and cultural stereotypes. Let us bear in mind the dictum of the great French physiologist Claude Bernard, who said, "That which we know is a great hindrance to our learning that which is as yet unknown."

AN EYEWITNESS ACCOUNT OF PAVLOV:

THE MAN, THE SCIENTIST AND HIS CONTRIBUTIONS
TO PSYCHOPHYSIOLOGY AND PSYCHIATRY

W. Horsley Gantt

Pavlovian Laboratory, VA Hospital
Perry Point, Maryland;
Department of Psychiatry, University of Maryland
Baltimore, Maryland

INTRODUCTION

The fate of men and of nations often depends upon accidents. For me to meet Pavlov on 28 October 1922, while working as a young doctor with the American Relief Administration in Petrograd [Leningrad], was an accident, but it was an act of free will that I stayed in Russia six more years to continue research with him. My sojourn was animated by an awe and respect for Pavlov, the creator of a quantitative science of behavior and a man whose courage and search for truth place him among the immortals.

When I went to the USSR in 1922, I had never heard of the conditional reflex; now every high school student has some familiarity with it. Today, 40 years after Pavlov's death (1936) at the age of 86, we witness the prophecy of H. G. Wells, writing in the New York Times in 1927, that the name of Pavlov would be much better known 100 years after his death than during his life.

To analyze why this is so would require another article. Perhaps telling why I remained in the USSR six years and learned the Russian language to work with him may give a clue. My contact with psychiatric literature and my frustration with the promises of Freud to give a satisfactory explanation for psychoses and neuroses made Pavlov's objective explanations welcome. He brilliantly demonstrated that the complex, so-called psychical phenomena of the dog could

5

be resolved into two events--the positive and the negative conditional reflexes--which can be measured quantitatively. Although in this procedure we do not have the complete answer to mental life, it was a major step in the development of the science of higher nervous activity.

BACKGROUND

The idea of reflex in its modern form can be traced back to Descartes in the beginning of the 17th century. He outlined the behavior of animals on a mechanistic basis similar to the operation of machines, while considering the psychical life of the human different from that of animals. The pineal gland, owing to its central and singular position, was assumed to make contact with the soul. Following Descartes' brilliant schemes was John Locke, who conceived of the individual as a tabula rasa whose record was written by the external environment during ontogenetic development. The importance of the external environment in behavior was further strengthened by Bell and Magendie's discovery of the neural basis for reflex function in the anterior and posterior nerve roots. The emphasis on the predominance of the external environment over the internal (including the subjective) was developed further by Condorcet and Helvetius, reaching its acme probably in Watson and Skinner. Pavlov's conditional reflex (CR), because of its quantitative, strictly physiological measurements, furnished an enormous impetus to behaviorism. In spite of Pavlov's attention to what went on inside the nervous system, the chief emphasis since Pavlov has been on the external environment.

The secret of Pavlov's success was his development of an objective method based on physiology. He had already completed his "Work of the Digestive Glands," winning the Nobel Prize in 1903, in which he described the conditional reflex and the method of producing it. His advance in physiology was due largely to his substitution of the chronic experiment for the former acute experiment, enabling him to study the animal over a long period of its life and to observe developments in its behavior related to the external environment.

The original discovery was the result of an accident: the observation that gastric secretion occurred when food was presented but before it was actually taken by the dog.

This observation was made possible by Pavlov's perfection of the Pavlovian pouch, through which he could collect gastric juice uncontaminated by food. In the course of feeding the animal daily, Pavlov noted that the gastric secretion began with the onset of the signals, <u>before</u> the animal actually received the food, e.g., to the appearance of the <u>Diener</u> (laboratory assistant), and even to his footsteps.

After two years' deliberation as to whether he should continue the study of this so-called psychical secretion, Pavlov perfected the method of separating the dog from adventitious stimuli of the external environment, using only the signals that he had selected. Employing salivary secretion as a quantitative measure for the conditional reflex, Pavlov developed an objective science for the study of conditioned excitation and conditioned inhibition. The inhibitory conditional reflex developed from the excitatory by failing to reinforce the original signal or a related one with food.

Using gastric or salivary secretion as an index of a conditional reflex, Pavlov found it impossible to obtain a quantitative measure of inhibition, since secretion could not fall below zero. Therefore, estimations of the intensity of inhibition were deduced by the effect of the inhibitory signals on aspects of behavior, e.g., sleep and various disturbances, as well as those which Pavlov called experimental neuroses.

Preceding the appearance of the <u>experimental neurosis</u> (a term used by Pavlov to cover all degrees of disturbed behavior, some of which would be termed psychotic by psychiatrists) were the <u>paradoxical</u> phases, viz., changed relationships among the excitatory conditional reflexes measured by their intensities, and also the relation of the intensity of the excitatory to the inhibitory conditional reflex. Pavlov noted that the paradoxical phases occurred when the animal was under stress.

These phases have been elaborated by the English psychiatrist Will Sargant (1957) as a basis for a number of pathological states, such as brainwashing, hysteria, conversions. Sargant considers that the abnormal behavior of the human with great emotional excitement, whether positive as in joy or negative as with pain, fear, or suppression,

leads to the perverse states similar to what Pavlov saw in
his dogs. People who show reversals of their behavior in
prisons or in excessively stimulating new situations are
thought by Sargant to be in the paradoxical phases. The
paradoxical phases might possible explain the behavior of
political prisoners exposed to isolation and various aversive, stressful stimuli, wherein normal behavior may be reversed, inhibition being converted into excitation.

Like the production of experimental neurosis by the
conflict of excitation and inhibition, the relation of the
paradoxical phases to neurosis is an interesting extension
of Pavlovian ideas; its applicability to the human, however,
requires more research.

As far back as 1925, Pavlov postulated the existence
of biochemical substances in the brain responsible for excitation and for inhibition. This was several years before
the discovery of acetylcholine by Loewi.

The ability of Pavlov to see new principles by careful
observation was exemplified not only in the original discovery in 1900 of the conditional reflex, but also in 1925
by observing the disturbances in various dogs occasioned by
a tidal flood in Leningrad during which they were trans-
ferred to new and strange quarters. Seeing that under the
same external conditions different animals became neurotic
in varying degrees, Pavlov postulated for his dogs a typology based on the Hippocratic four temperaments--two central
and normal: 1) sanguine and 2) phlegmatic, and two extreme
and pathological: 3) manic (excitatory) and 4) melancholic
(inhibitory). Although up to this time it has not been possible to find a strict and satisfactory basis for typology,
the importance of Pavlov's typology was his recognition that
internal differences in the animals were responsible for
their behavior. Thus, Pavlov departed from strict dependence
on the external environment and included constitutional or
genetic factors. Just as Pavlov had in his earlier experiments looked within the nervous system trying to discover
principles, here he postulated also internal differences
(Pavlov, 1928, pp. 370-378).

Pavlov's science has differed from American psychology
not only in the methods of what is now called classical and
operant conditioning but in the number of theories he pro-

posed for what went on within the nervous system. The advantage of Skinner's adhering to factual measures of what
occurred on the surface, although too limited, is that he
has substituted data for a welter of unverified assumptions
common to psychiatry. Pavlov's enunciation of theory was
more than fanciful in that he usually devised critical experiments for verification.

Another important inclusion in Pavlov's system was his
attention to language in the human. This function he thought
rested upon the ability of the human to form long chains of
conditional reflexes through words, i.e., for generalization
and abstract thinking. In spite of the characterization of
the human as differing from the subhuman in the function
represented by language, implicit as well as explicit,
Pavlov himself contributed very little to the further development of the idea; this was probably due to his age--
over 80 at the time of this concept.

After his 80th year, Pavlov attempted to apply his
ideas to the psychiatric clinic, using his concepts of protective inhibition, which he considered a factor in schizophrenia. This psychosis, in his thinking, depended upon the
principle which he saw in his dogs of excessive stimulation
through increasing intensity of conditional signals passing
over into inhibition. In spite of some years of attempted
therapeutic application of this idea in the USSR after
Pavlov's death, it seems to be of little value (Pavlov,
1941, pp. 78-80).

PAVLOV'S SUCCESSORS

In the USSR, several of Pavlov's pupils (Anokhin,
Asratyan, Kreps, Kupalov) have been prominent in extending
his work. Of these, the only survivors are Kreps and Asratyan; for the latter there has been built a large institute
in Moscow employing 650 people for the investigation of conditional reflexes. (The third surviving pupil of Pavlov is
the author of this article.) Anokhin's concepts and researches have been translated by Corson and published in
this country in an impressive volume (Anokhin, 1974).

Anokhin had during Pavlov's life attacked the problem
of the relationship between the periphery and the center

through the transplantation of nerves (brachial to vagus),
electrophysiology, the formatio reticularis, etc. Kupalov
continued Pavlov's researches at the Institute of Experimental Medicine in Leningrad where Pavlov did most of his
experiments after 1900. Kupalov introduced the idea of the
difference between the dog on the stand and the dog allowed
to run freely in a large room. Kupalov's chief pupil, now
Director of the Institute of Experimental Medicine, is
M. M. Khananashvili, author of several important books. He
has further developed Kupalov's ideas, as well as expanded
the concept of schizokinesis. He introduced the idea of
informational neurosis due to crowding too much information
into a short time. Orbeli, another prominent pupil of Pavlov
who died a decade ago, has left a prominent pupil, E. M.
Kreps, the Director of the Genetic Institute in Leningrad.
Krasnogorsky, an early pupil of Pavlov's, and Ivanov-
Smolensky applied the conditional reflex method to the study
of children; in his later life Krasnogorsky did considerable
work on the formation of language in children.

My own researches differ from the Russian studies in
that I have devoted more attention to the analysis and limitations of the formation of the conditional reflex. Since I
am more familiar with my own work than with that of others,
I shall devote more space to its description.

Pavlov, the pioneer, had a greater interest and enthusiasm in extending the horizon of the conditional reflex
and developing the concept that this was the real scientific
basis of behavior. Although Pavlov was careful to separate
the functions of unconditional and conditional reflexes and
to rely on experimental data, he felt that nearly all visceral phenomena could become conditional reflexes. With his
dynamic ebullience he was more concerned with this extensive
view rather than with its restrictive limitations. Pavlov
shared the enthusiasm of the 19th-century scientists who en-
visioned the omnipotence of the scientific method which had
been stated by Francis Bacon 300 years earlier: "Knowledge
is power." Pavlov did not live long enough to become frustrated with the attainments of science as did Born, Einstein,
Aldous Huxley and some others who saw the destructive uses
to which science was put. Thus, Born and Einstein expressed
doubts as to the positive value of science and hesitated to
say whether they would, with this hindsight, become scientists if they had their lives to live over. It is likely,

however, that Pavlov, owing to his positive, dynamic nature, would never have become disillusioned but would have sought to find the positive application of his science. He took pains, however, to vociferate against Marxist claims of re-making the individual by saying that Marxism did not distinguish between the unmodifiable part of human nature, i.e., the unconditional reflex, and that which would be changed by environment, the conditional reflex. With equal justification he might have objected to the exclusive materialistic philosophy (if it can be dignified by this term) of behaviorism everywhere, especially in the USA; indeed, he had clearly averred the importance of the subjective, but he said science could study only the objective (Pavlov, 1928, pp. 80-128).

In the following paragraphs I shall describe my extensions of Pavlov's ideas, the limitations of the possibility for conditional reflex formation, the additional principles which I have found in experimental neurosis, and several new concepts described by the terms autokinesis, schizokinesis, centrokinesis and organ-system responsibility. I shall also say a word about my concept of the subjective and the internal universe.

EXPERIMENTAL NEUROSIS

In 1922, Pavlov observed that confronted with a discrimination between positive and negative conditional reflexes to food--where the conditional stimuli were very similar, e.g., two tones close together in pitch--the dogs became disturbed to varying degrees. All of these states, whether neurotic or psychotic, he called experimental neuroses. Later he saw that the appearance and nature of the neurosis depended upon the type of dog. He postulated that in susceptible dogs similar stimuli involving excitation and inhibition impinged onto adjacent areas of the brain and that the chemical substances underlying excitation and inhibition were brought too closely together. Pavlov also described pathological stages of the developing neurosis which he called paradoxical and in extreme cases ultraparadoxical and inhibitory. In these phases the conditional reflexes, which had been graded in their intensities, became of equal intensity (paradoxical) or even reversed in their intensities, so that the formerly weaker ones became the

stronger (ultraparadoxical). In the last phase all conditional reflexes became inhibitory (Pavlov, 1928, pp. 344-366).

In my studies of several dogs throughout their lives,
from puppyhood to their deaths in the laboratory at 14-18
years of age, I was able to trace the neuroses over long
periods and to see principles which could not bee seen over
a shorter period. I shall enumerate these briefly.

It appeared to me that the difficult differentiation
between sensory stimuli was not the major cause of the neuroses and that much more important were the relations of
the dog to the experimenter, which I later called Effect of
Person. This force, Effect of Person, though a general one
in all dogs, normal and pathological, was much greater in
the pathological dogs. The Person could become a disturbing
influence or, on the other hand, a palliative one. The presence of the Person often produced all the neurotic symptoms
seen during difficult differentiation; but on the contrary,
certain relationships of the Person, such as petting the
dog, ameliorated or removed entirely the symptoms during the
petting. Here was a marked ambivalence (Gantt et al, 1966).

Later I recognized the Effect of Person not only as a
force between dog and experimenter but as existing throughout the animal kingdom from one individual to another, extending from the human down to insects. By the term Effect
of Person, I intend to convey the idea of the effect of any
individual on another individual, whether man on dog, dog on
dog, or insect on insect. This is a complex force depending
both upon inborn and upon acquired characteristics. As every
psychiatrist and every physician knows, it is an effective
adjunct to therapy; on the other hand, it may be destructive.

In my prolonged study of experimental neurosis, I also
saw that many physiological systems became involved, that
the original focus of disturbance (in the food center)
spread to include many other physiological systems, e.g.,
respiratory, cardiovascular, genitourinary, and metabolic.
The study of sexual phenomena, which range from extreme inhibitory (impotentia) to excessive excitatory (ejaculatio
praecox), showed that the production of sexual symptoms in
the dog may arise on the basis of simple extension of the
pathological focus to involve many systems and that it may
be a generalized spread rather than arising from a specific

focus originally in the sexual center, in contradistinction
to Freud's postulates.

The cardiovascular system has been studied systematically by my collaborators and me since 1939, when I firmly
established the cardiac conditional reflex. Later we demonstrated (Dykman and Gantt, 1960) that changes in blood
pressure could become conditional reflexes and that these
hypertensive reflexes could persist for years. Newton further showed in the Pavlovian laboratory that coronary blood
flow to conditional signals and Person could exceed the
coronary blood flow to the eating of food.

The addition of cardiovascular function as a component
of the conditional reflex indicated that other visceral systems beyond the gastrointestinal, with which Pavlov began,
could readily become conditioned. It has not been sufficiently recognized--and often forgotten in this country--
that Pavlov began and did most of his work with the autonomic nervous functions. In the USA operant conditioning
was formerly done with the motor system. In the past decade
this method has been applied to autonomic functions, as if
autonomic conditioning were a new discovery.

The prolonged study of dogs, often for their whole
lives, and the comparison of several components of the
conditional reflex (cardiovascular, respiratory, motor,
secretory) revealed differences among these components--
differences in the speed of formation and in the resistance
to extinction. Although cardiovascular functions (heart
rate, blood pressure) often formed after one reinforcement
by the unconditional stimulus (food, shock), paradoxically
this function would persist in the face of extinction, while
the secretory and motor components dropped out. It appeared
that the general supporting functions, e.g., the respiratory
and the cardiovascular, were quick to form and slow to disappear, while the specific functions (secretion, movement)
were slower to form but extinguished more rapidly. To this
difference in rate of formation and of extinction we gave
the name schizokinesis. This phenomenon seemed to me to
represent a constitutional dysharmony in the organism,
which in an exaggerated form was a basis for neurotic development (Gantt, 1953).

Conditioning studies on renal function have been carried out extensively by Bykov in the USSR and by Corson in the USA. Contrary to Bykov's claims of a precise conditional diuresis with dual control, hormonal and vascular, my prolonged studies in dogs with the kidney in situ, as well as in those dogs in which the kidney was transplanted to the neck to eliminate the renal nerves, demonstrated the lack of formation of a positive conditional renal reflex (increased diuresis in response to signals for drinking water). Corson also could not duplicate the findings of Bykov, although he described conditional antidiuretic responses (Corson, 1966).

From more than a decade of work with a number of dogs with renal fistulae, comparing the results with the conditionability of other organs such as the gastrointestinal and the cardiovascular, a new principle appeared, that of organ-system responsibility (Gantt, 1972, 1974). My understanding of the various organs in the body is that each one has a special function to perform and that whether this function can become a conditional reflex depends upon the role of the function in the body economy. That such functions as salivary and gastric secretions and changes in heart rate and blood flow, as well as in respiration, should be conditionable is teleological and homeostatic because these organs have to perform a function quickly to meet the emergency demands of the organism. Furthermore, in the fluctuating situations of life, where the results are highly variable, sometimes proceeding regularly where the signal is followed by the usual event and sometimes where the signal is not thus followed, there is nothing lost to the economy in the latter case except a small amount of energy needed to increase heart rate or to produce secretion. The contents, electrolytes, etc., of the secretions are not lost to the organism, because the secretions remain within the alimentary tract until they are reabsorbed into the system.

However, the situation is entirely different with the secretion of urine; whatever fluid passes into the pelvis of the kidney is forever lost to the organism because it cannot be reabsorbed either from the renal pelvis or from the bladder and on reaching these receptacles it is essentially on the outside of the body. If the kidney were to secrete large amounts of water, electrolytes, and other necessary substances simply to signals, it might be depleting the body of much needed substances and upsetting normal homeostasis.

This organ-system responsibility seems to be a principle operating not only with the kidney but throughout the
organism; it is a function designed to keep the organism in
balance and to prevent the vacillations that might be caused
by conditional reflex formation which could never be of any
teleological value. A comparison of the functions of the
kidney with those of the gastrointestinal and cardiovascular
systems will emphasize that these organs have very different
functions to perform in the body economy: a conditional reflex in one physiological system will be in the main (though
not in all instances) useful and preserving of life; in the
other it would perhaps never be useful and could be destructive.

AUTOKINESIS

In the study of the individual over its life span, and
especially in the neurotic dogs, we saw the appearance of
new symptoms referable to the old situations but which developed after the dogs were removed from the environment
which produced the disturbance. In the pathological animals
this development was a negative one, i.e., one which added
to the pathology of the animal. It was thus apparent that
there were pathological developing processes occurring, while
nothing was being done to the dog, but based on the traces in
the nervous sytem of what had been done. This phenomenon I
called autokinesis. Well-known to all physicians is an opposite type of autokinesis, i.e., an improvement based on
a short period of contact with the physician or of psychotherapy. This kind of development in individuals referable
to one experience which produces a life-long improvement of
functioning in the individual, and the process of simple development in the organism, is of such common occurrence that
we tend to overlook it as we do the force of gravitation
because we are constantly surrounded by it.

Autokinesis can thus be either beneficial (positive)
or destructive (negative).

Autokinesis can be shown in some cases to be based on
anatomical changes such as those revealed by Jerzy Rose,
who showed that cortical cells will put out new processes
to make connections with other cells across a destroyed
layer of the cortex, and it has been postulated by Eccles

(1975) that in old age, although there may be a loss of
millions of neurons, new processes grow from the remaining
cells to make new connections with other cells.

These phenomena, to which I give the general terms of
positive or negative autokinesis, have been described recently as neural plasticity by Hans Lucas-Teuber.

CENTROKINESIS

Another related problem to which I have devoted considerable attention is: What principles determine whether
the effects of an agent can become conditioned? My interest
evolved from a desire to analyze critically the laws of conditioning, to know if every physiological function of the
organism is conditionable. Some early work had been done in
the USA, showing that responses produced by peripheral stimulation at the nerve ending, e.g., the action of pilocarpine
in producing salivary secretion, could not become conditioned, while salivary secretion to food was the beginning
of Pavlov's work on the conditional reflex.

Choosing a drug (pilocarpine) to produce hyperglycemia
because this effect had been shown by Brooks (1931) to occur
by direct action on the tissues not involving the central
nervous system, Gantt et al (1937) were unable to see any
conditioning of hyperglycemia, although the same hyperglycemia to fear had been reported as conditionable. This phenomenon I have recently called centrokinesis (Gantt, 1972,
1974).

SUBJECTIVE AND OBJECTIVE

I am in agreement with Pavlov's decision to eliminate
subjective explanations in the study of behavior and to remain
on an objective basis as well as with his qualifying statement that we are chiefly concerned with our subjective life.
Moreover, I feel that we should not minimize in our separation of objective and subjective the recognition of the subjective, and that we must separate the questions that science can answer from those to which it can give no answer.
Pavlov, who made his great contributions by devising an
objective experiment giving quantitative measures (units

of secretion), also spoke of the importance of duty, moral
responsibility and his belief in free will (Pavlov, 1941,
p. 144).

BIBLIOGRAPHY

ANOKHIN, P. K. (1974). Biology and Neurophysiology of the
    Conditioned Reflex and its Role in Adaptive Behavior.
    Trans. and ed. by S. A. Corson, Pergamon Press, New
    York.

BROOKS, C. M. (1931). A delimitation of the central nervous
    mechanism involved in reflex hyperglycemia. Am. J.
    Physiol. 99:64-76.

CORSON, S. A. (1966). Conditioning of water and electrolyte
    excretion. In: Endocrines and the Central Nervous Sys-
    tem, ed. by Rachmiel Levine, Williams & Wilkins, Bal-
    timore, pp. 140-199.

DYKMAN, R. A. and W. H. GANTT (1960). Experimental psycho-
    genic hypertension: Blood pressure changes conditioned
    to painful stimuli (Schizokinesis). Bull. Johns Hop-
    kins Hosp., 107(2).

ECCLES, J. C. (1975). Reported in lecture by Hans Lucas-
    Teuber, Johns Hopkins University, December 1975.

GANTT, W. H. (1953). Principles of nervous breakdown-
    schizokinesis and autokinesis. Ann. N.Y. Acad. Sci.,
    56(2).

GANTT, W. H. (1972). Organ-system responsibility, homeo-
    stasis and the conditional reflex. Cond. Ref., 7(1).

GANTT, W. H. (1974). Autokinesis, schizokinesis, centro-
    kinesis and organ-system responsibility: Concepts and
    definition. Pav. J. Biol. Sci., 9(4).

GANTT, W. H., S. KATZENELBOGEN, and R. B. LOUCKS (1937).
    An attempt to condition adrenalin hyperglycemia. Bull.
    Johns Hopkins Hosp., LX(6).

GANTT, W. H., J. E. O. NEWTON, F. L. ROYER, and J. H.
    STEPHENS (1966). Effect of person. Cond. Ref., 1(1).

PAVLOV, I. P. (1928). Lectures on Conditional Reflexes.
    Trans. and ed. by W. Horsley Gantt, Internat. Pub.,
    New York.

PAVLOV, I. P. (1941). Conditioned Reflexes and Psychiatry.
    Trans. and ed. by W. Horsley Gantt, Internat. Pub.,
    New York.

SARGANT, W. (1957). Battle for the Mind. Doubleday Co.,
    New York.

PHILOSOPHICAL AND HISTORICAL ROOTS OF

PAVLOVIAN PSYCHOBIOLOGY*

Samuel A. Corson and Elizabeth O'Leary Corson

Department of Psychiatry

The Ohio State University, Columbus, Ohio

I. PROLOGUE

Perhaps the most distinguishing characteristic of Pavlovian psychobiology is the holistic integrated approach to the study of living systems and the recognition of the central role of the nervous system in the maintenance of biological homeostasis in higher organisms. This holistic approach has been referred to in Russian biomedical literature as the theory of "nervism" or the neurogenic theory. This theory emphasizes the concept of the organism as a whole, the leading role of the cerebral cortex in the regulation of physiologic and behavioral homeostasis, and the importance of psychosocial factors in health and disease.

The development of the neurogenic theory of integrative psychobiology is generally ascribed to two Russian scientists: the physiologist Ivan Mikhailovich Sechenov (1829-1905) and the clinician Sergei Petrovich Botkin (1832-1889). Sechenov's contribution to the theory of nervism was given its most definitive formulation in his monograph Reflexes of the Brain (Sechenov, 1863) in which he stated that: "all acts of conscious or unconscious life in their origin are reflexes."

*The research work of the authors was supported in part by grants from The Commonwealth Fund, USPHS grants NB 04769, NBLM 05006, LM 00635, MH 12089, MH 18098, the Foundations' Fund for Research in Psychiatry, The Rockefeller Brothers Fund, The Central Ohio Heart Assoc., the Ohio State University Graduate School Biomedical Research Support Grant, and the Grant Foundation.

It is interesting that the original title Sechenov had chosen for his book was: An Attempt to Introduce a Physiological Basis for Psychological Processes . Under pressure from the tsarist censor, Sechenov was obliged to change the title to Reflexes of the Brain.

Sergei Petrovich Botkin was Professor of Internal Medicine at the Petersburg Medico-Surgical Academy in which Sechenov was, for a time, Professor of Physiology. Botkin was a physiologically oriented clinician who had the imagination and audacity to organize in his clinic in 1861 the first clinical laboratory which he personally directed until 1878, when he delegated the direction of the laboratory to Ivan Petrovich Pavlov. Pavlov remained as head of that laboratory for ten years. In addition to routine clinical laboratory work, Pavlov, together with Botkin, undertook the development of physiological experiments on animals, working primarily on the physiology of the cardiovascular system. It was during that period that Pavlov made the important discovery of the role of the sympathetic nervous system in the regulation of cardiac function.

Credit for the development of the principles of biological integration should also go to Claude Bernard (1859, 1865), who elaborated the concept of the constancy of the internal environment of living organisms. Although the state of biochemistry in Bernard's time could offer only a meagre insight into the complex composition and architecture of the internal environment of living systems, nevertheless, Bernard had the imagination to formulate the concept of biochemical homeostasis which was later abundantly confirmed by careful experimentation.

Claude Bernard formulated his concept as follows:

> Animals have really two environments:
> a milieu extérieur...and a milieu
> intérieur in which the tissue elements
> live. The living organism does not
> really exist in the milieu extérieur...
> but in the liquid milieu intérieur formed
> by the circulating organic liquid which
> surrounds and bathes all the tissue ele-
> ments...This milieu intérieur never
> changes, atmospheric fluctuations can not
> penetrate beyond its boundaries and,
> therefore, one may confidently state that

> the physiological conditions of the
> internal medium in higher organisms
> are constant...The organism is en-
> closed in a sort of hothouse...All
> physiologic mechanisms...have only
> one aim--the preservation of constant
> conditions of life within the inter-
> nal phase.

Sechenov (1861), who was primarily interested in the
central nervous system and in the interaction of the organism with the external environment, insisted that:

> an organism without the external medium
> which supports its existence is impos-
> sible. Therefore, in the scientific
> description of an organism one must in-
> clude also the medium which exerts in-
> fluence on it...The idea that an organ-
> ism is a body that includes within it-
> self conditions required for its
> existence is false and harmful.

This divergence of viewpoints appeared to be a result
of a failure of communication and is perhaps symbolic of
the persistent philosophical cleavage between the East and
the West. Actually Claude Bernard did not mean to imply
that higher organisms are statically insulated from, and
have no interchange with, their external environment. In
his book, An Introduction to the Study of Experimental
Medicine, Bernard (1865, p. 75) clearly states his views:

> The conditions necessary to life are
> found neither in the organism nor in the
> outer environment, but in both at once.
> Indeed, if we suppress or disturb the
> organism, life ceases, even though the
> environment remains intact; if, on the
> other hand, we take away or vitiate the
> environment, life just as completely
> disappears, even though the organism has
> not been destroyed...In the same way,
> life results from contact of the organism
> with its environment; we can no more
> understand it through the organism alone
> than the environment alone.

This lack of communication is particularly strange, since Sechenov worked in Bernard's laboratory during the academic year of 1862. It was there that Sechenov performed his famous experiment on frogs, wherein he demonstrated for the first time the principle of central inhibition, a discovery of major significance for neurophysiology and psychology. Yet Bernard apparently exhibited as singular a lack of appreciation of the importance of Sechenov's discovery as Sechenov did for Bernard's formulation of the principle of internal homeostasis.

The concept of the constancy of the internal biological environment ranks in importance with the theory of organic evolution. What Claude Bernard pointed out was that biological processes can proceed only within a rather narrow range of physico-chemical factors. The ability of higher organisms to maintain their own constant internal climate endowed them with a certain degree of independence and freedom from the external milieu and thus made it possible for them to survive in a wide variety of environments in which lower organisms would perish.

Similarly, Sechenov's discovery of central inhibition and his pioneering attempts at formulating a physiological basis for behavior, culminating in his monumental treatise on Reflexes of the Brain (Sechenov, 1863), represented a scientific event of major significance, an achievement in which Bernard should have taken pride, since the initial discovery of central inhibition was made by Sechenov in Bernard's laboratory. Yet, in Bernard's publications there appears to be no mention of Sechenov's contributions to physiology; nor have I been able to discover in Sechenov's writings an appreciation of, or even any reference to, Bernard's principle of internal homeostasis.

This seemingly studied neglect of Bernard's major contribution was apparent even in the scholarly and generally all-inclusive Russian thirty-six volume Large Medical Encyclopedia. In a contribution by V. Shidlovskii (1957), Claude Bernard's work is described in detail, but no mention is made of his concept of the constancy of the internal biological medium. Considering the fact that subsequent careful biochemical investigations proved the correctness of Bernard's concept and that this idea probably represented the first intimation of the principles of biological cybernetics, such an omission seems to be strange indeed. The only time I encountered in the Russian literature a reference to Bernard's formulation of internal homeostasis was in a recent monograph by Ginetsinskii (1963), and in an erudite article by Lisitsyn (1961) in the Bol'shaya Medits-inskaya Entsiklopediya on the theory of nervism in which Lisitsyn pointed out that Bernard was fully aware of the role of the nervous system in the integration of biological functions.

The neglect of Sechenov's contributions to neurophysiology and to the behavioral sciences in the English scientific literature is equally glaring and consistent. Until recently, Sechenov's name has not been mentioned in American or English textbooks of physiology, psychology, or psychiatry; not even in John F. Fulton's (1949 b) Physiology of the Nervous System, in spite of the fact that Fulton was one of the first American neurophysiologists who had a deep appreciation of the contributions of the Russian School of integrative physiology. The first American reference to Sechenov's book appears to be by Mary Brazier (1959) in an historical introduction to the Handbook of Physiology.

This lack of rapport cannot be ascribed entirely to linguistic differences. The barrier is due primarily to a fundamental divergence of philosophical orientation. This basic cleavage has been particularly glaring in the case of psychiatry and psychology. The superimposition of political overtones in the East and in the West, and the continuing presence of a linguistic barrier contributed no little to the perpetuation of disharmony and misunderstanding and hindered the development of meaningful communication. During the past two decades, particularly since the advent of the Sputnik era, some avenues of linguistic and philosophic communication did open up. However, thus far there have been few systematic attempts to develop a continuous dialogue in the spirit of friendly, objective scientific inquiry.

Walter B. Cannon (1929, 1932) expanded and furnished brilliant experimental verification for Bernard's postulates by demonstrating the operation of a number of physiologic and endocrine mechanisms by means of which living organisms maintain physiologic and biochemical homeostasis, a term coined by Cannon.

W. Horsley Gantt (1944, 1953, 1960, 1962) made major
significant contributions in this area not only by his
masterful translations of Pavlov's works (1928, 1941), but
also by his extensive original experimental studies, especially on conditional cardiac responses. Gantt's formulation of the principles of schizokinesis and autokinesis
represents a milestone in the development of a scientific
basis for psychosomatic and cerebrovisceral medicine.

II. PHILOSOPHICAL MATERIALISM, VITALISM, AND MECHANISTIC
     REDUCTIONISM. THE MIND-BRAIN DICHOTOMY VERSUS A
     HOLISTIC APPROACH IN PSYCHOBIOLOGY AND MEDICINE

Pavlovian psychobiology is based on the assumption that
no cleavage or separation is possible between mind and body
(or between mind and brain) no more than it is feasible to
separate locomotion from the muscles or circulation from the
cardiovascular system. The brain is the organ of the mind;
the central nervous system represents the physicochemical
basis of learning, emotions, and all behavior. According to
Pavlovian theory, mental and emotional processes are considered to be a result of the function of the brain in the integration of the reflex activities of the internal and external environments of the organism. The brain is looked
upon as an organ of information-gathering, storage, and retrieval, its activity thus leading to the development of a
subjective image of objective reality. The correct reflection of the objective world (i.e., reality testing) enables
the organism to adjust its activities to the demands of the
environment and thus to develop adaptive behavior.

In considering the external milieu, the Pavlovian
school assigns an important role to the social components of
the environment in molding the behavior of man. The unitary
theory of the brain-mind-social environment complex represents the quintessence of the Pavlovian school. Perhaps an
apt description for this trend in psychiatric thinking would
be cerebrosocial psychiatry.

This cleavage in the approach to psychophysiologic
disturbances is in reality not merely a difference between
the East and the West, but is basically a difference between
the orientation of most experimental scientists and the proponents of philosophical idealism and mind-body dualism.

Homer W. Smith (1953, 1959), one of America's most creative and erudite physiologists, elegantly summarized this philosophical cleavage:

> This Cartesian dichotomy between 'matter' and 'mind' lingers on, not only in common parlance but in philosophy, giving rise to frequent discussions of the 'mind-brain problem' or the 'mind-body problem'. Some critical thinkers continue to adhere to dualism, holding to the belief in something called 'mind' which is other than matter, but the majority of workers in the biological sciences reject the belief in the existence of disembodied mind and see in 'mind' a mode or property of matter, so that psychical processes are wholly dependent on physical and chemical events in the nervous system. This philosophical position is commonly identified as 'materialism', but the term 'naturalism' is to be preferred--because the ultimate nature of matter and energy remain unknown, and the task of science and philosophy is to study nature as given, and without prejudicial preconceptions.

It is instructive to observe the similarity of the brain-mind concept developed by I. P. Pavlov and by John F. Fulton. Pavlov (1903, 1951) expressed this as follows:

> The time is coming, and it surely will come, when there will occur a natural and inevitable rapprochement, and finally an amalgamation, of the psychologic and the physiologic, the subjective and the objective; the problem, that for such a long time troubled human thought, will be experimentally solved.

Fulton (1949 a, p. 101), commenting in his own inimitable, generous, and constructive manner on Sherrington's dualism, put it this way:

Sir Charles Sherrington in his Foreword
to the 1947 edition of The Integrative Action
of the Nervous System states his belief that
man is no farther along to-day in accounting
for mental processes in physiological terms
than was Aristotle two thousand years ago.
A similar thought was expressed in his Rede
Lecture of 1933, quoted at the beginning of
this volume. 'What right', he asked, 'have
we to conjoin mental experience with physiological? No scientific right, only the right
of what Keats, with that superlative Shakes-
pearian gift of his, dubbed "busy common
sense".' There are many who would take issue
with Sir Charles's conservative pronouncement,
for the more one reads of Sherrington's own
writings, the more evident it becomes that
he himself has pointed the way which will
ultimately lead to a sound interpretation
of the mind-body relationship. I believe,
too, that the lobotomist, if he studies his
patients as closely as Sherrington studied
his monkeys and chimpanzees, will one day
be in a position to interpret the brain as
the organ of the mind.

What elements of mentation led Sherrington and Pavlov
to such contradictory views regarding the nature of mental
activity would represent a good subject for the analysis of
the nature of thinking. One aspect of Sherrington's analysis
of the "mind" is indicated in his book, Man on His Nature
(1941). Sherrington was troubled by the fact that the "mind"
unlike the body, appears to be biologically discontinuous or
"phasic", i.e., it appears only at a certain stage in the
development of a human being. As pointed out by Homer Smith
(1953, 1959):

Sherrington's difficulty arose in part from
his persistence in the use of the word 'mind'
in the Cartesian sense: as 'something that
exists' in the sense in which matter and
energy exist. Long ago the philosopher
David Hume (1896) defined 'mind' as an abstract term denoting the series of ideas,
memories, and feelings which appear in consciousness, and which so overlap that they

give the impression of being continuous...
There is no more warrant for speaking of
this temporal sequence as a 'thing' than
of so describing the <u>sequence</u> of flicker-
ing images that appear on the cinema.

The pivotal point that separated the orientation of
Sherrington, Claude Bernard and Sigmund Freud from that of
the Sechenov-Botkin-Pavlov school is the adherence of the
former to <u>mechanistic concepts</u> in biology. The onset of the
Industrial Revolution and the glorification of the machine
in the West hastened the development of scientific biology
and the decline of vitalistic trends in biomedical thinking.
Biologists began to think of living organisms as machines,
subject to the same laws of physics and chemistry that gov-
ern inanimate objects.

A logical outgrowth of this orientation was the development of the anatomic localistic cellular-organ theory of
disease, propounded particularly by Virchow (1858) in his
<u>Cellular Pathology</u>. Disease was thought of as being due to
highly circumscribed, localized disturbances in specific
tissues, by analogy with man-made machines. Similarly,
therapy was considered chiefly in terms of repair of specific
tissues or organs.

This reductionist mechanistic trend in biomedical sciences laid the background for the detailed studies of the
functions of various organs and cells. This served as a
basis for the development of rational methods for diagnosis
and therapy. However, this investigative-therapeutic system
<u>failed to take into consideration the integrative adaptive
aspects of the organism as a whole</u>. Consequently it led its
proponents into therapeutic errors and philosophical difficulties.

In diagnosis and therapy, this system failed to pay
sufficient attention to the importance of psychologic and
environmental factors. Philosophically, those who attempted
to apply mechanistically the laws of physics and chemistry
to biological systems were eventually driven back to vitalism
when they attempted to study mental and emotional problems,
because the known physicochemical laws could not explain
biological integration and behavioral phenomena. That appears
to be one reason why Claude Bernard and Sherrington shied away
from studying higher integrating functions of the brain.

In contrast to the mechanistic approach of the Virchow school,* Russian biomedical thinking, even before the advent of Sechenov, Botkin, and Pavlov, developed chiefly on the basis of holistic integrative concepts (see Corson, 1957). It is conceivable that the persistence of a primitive agrarian economy in Russia and the relative absence of man-made machines may have contributed to this holistic organismic approach.

Another factor that may have contributed to the philosophic sophistication of Russian biomedical scientists and clinicians was the development of extensive intimate contacts with liberal intellectuals in other areas of endeavor. Sechenov, the physiologist, and Botkin, the clinician, were strongly influenced in their thinking by such philosophers and literary critics as N. G. Chernyshevskii and A. I. Gertsen** (see Koshtoyants, 1946). Chernyshevskii (1860) published his erudite Anthropologic Principle in Philosophy in which he proposed a unitary theory of the organic and inorganic. He also elaborated the concept that specific configurations of chemical elements endow the new materials with new qualities. He reasoned that human consciousness can best be understood in terms of the historical (evolutionary) development of psychologic phenomena in the entire animal kingdom. Higher forms of psychologic function are thus expressions of the development of new and more complex patterns of configuration of matter. This philosophic orientation can be described as historical materialism in contrast to mechanistic materialism.

It is on the basis of this philosophic orientation that Sechenov and Botkin formulated the theory of nervism which laid the background for Pavlov's elaboration of the theory of conditional reflexes and which eventually gave birth to an integrative and systems approach in biomedical thinking.

---

*It should be pointed out here that in his later years, Virchow emphasized the importance of psychosocial factors in the maintenance of good health and prevention of disease. He even referred to medicine as a social science. See Virchow, 1958.

**Gertsen, A. I., 1812-1870, a distinguished Russian philosopher, writer, and revolutionary democrat. Known in Western publications as Herzen or Hertzen. He was the son of a wealthy Russian landlord, Ivan Alekseevich Yakovlev, and a German woman. Since this marriage was not formalized, the father gave his son the surname "Herzen" ("from the heart").

The essence of the theory of nervism (or the neurogenic theory of medicine) can be summarized as follows:

1. All living processes, including consciousness, can be ultimately analyzed in terms of natural laws. However, the specific configuration of materials forming living organisms endows them with properties not possessed by the individual components. The properties of H_2O or of H_2O_2 do not represent a mere summation of the properties of the component elements. A new quality is represented in a molecule of H_2O or of H_2O_2, this quality being determined by the specific configuration of the elements. The appearance of a new quality in a chemical compound does not compel the chemist to resort to mysticism in explaining the properties of water or of a tobacco mosaic virus molecule. By the same reasoning, a biologist need not invoke mystical vitalism to explain the properties of living matter. A biologist or a chemist could choose to resort to mysticism, but this type of approach fails to provide either understanding, prediction, or control.

2. Nature contains many hierarchies of levels of organization and configuration of matter, each level possessing characteristic qualities. The quality we call "life" appeared at a particular level of organization of certain material entities. Consciousness and mind are qualities characteristic for a certain level of organization of neural elements.

3. Living organisms are characterized by the presence of a hierarchy of different levels of integration, beginning with intracellular integration and leading up to integration of organs and organ systems by means of a central nervous system. In higher animals, the central nervous system itself is structured on the basis of integrated hierarchic levels, the cerebral cortex assuming a progressively increasing dominant role in animals higher in the evolutionary scale. Cerebrovisceral theory added the emphasis that this increase in cerebral dominance in higher animals also holds true for visceral and endocrine functions.

4. The progressively increasing dominance of the cerebral mantle in higher organisms, and especially in man, and the resulting increase in the multiplicity of physiologic responses to symbols of physicochemical stimuli, multiplied

the possibilities for the impingement of psychologic factors
on somatic and visceral functions. Consequently, the
Sechenov-Botkin-Pavlov neurogenic theory of medicine led to
the emphasis of the importance of psychosocial factors in
diagnosis, therapy and prophylaxis. Thus was prepared the
physiologic basis for psychosomatic medicine.

As an illustration of the practical application of the
theory of nervism, one may cite the clinical orientation of
S. P. Botkin (see Corson, 1957). For example, Botkin looked
upon fever as a defense mechanism (in which the central
nervous system played an important role) and did not encourage the excessive use of drugs in combating fevers, a
practice that was fashionable among medical circles at that
time. He advocated the use of drugs with care and only when
they were definitely indicated. Botkin suggested the need
for studying the mechanisms used by the organism in combating
disease:

> It is in this studying of the natural
> abortive forms (of disease), the learning
> of the methods used by the organism in
> combating infection, it appears to me,
> that we shall find that path that will
> lead us to the discovery of recuperating,
> disease-combating remedies.

Botkin urged that treatment be directed toward the patient
and not just toward a localized disease.

The direction of Pavlov's research on the psychic
aspects of gastrointestinal physiology and later on conditioned reflexes can be traced directly to the influence of
the ideas of Botkin. A number of Botkin's other students
continued to develop these therapeutic principles in their
clinical teaching and practice. One of these students,
V. A. Manassein, developed a keen insight into psychosomatic
factors in disease. He insisted that psychologic factors
not only can produce temporary disturbances in various visceral functions but may also lead to a host of chronic
diseases.

Manassein's remarks regarding hospital environments
(Manassein, 1876, pp. 141-148) could be read with profit by
many hospital administrators today.

> In this respect most hospitals and
> clinics present a very unhappy pic-
> ture with their unfriendly uniform
> wards and their dull monotonous
> daily routines. Such shameful con-
> ditions in our hospitals, in my
> opinion, are no less harmful to the
> patients than all the other errors in
> regard to hygienic and dietetic arrange-
> ments, thanks to which many patients
> perish, not because of their diseases,
> but because of their hospitals...

In such hospital environments

> the thoughts of patients have nothing
> to concentrate on...they are therefore
> invariably centered around their own
> pains...The first concern of a physician
> who understands the significance of psychic
> influences should be with the need for a
> more cozy appearance of the wards. In
> this respect, flower arrangements, birds
> in cages, wall pictures, aquaria, and so
> forth, would help us, without interfering
> with hygienic requirements of cleanliness
> and simplicity, to a large extent to re-
> move that uniform dishearteningly deadly
> character which reflects itself at pre-
> sent from almost every hospital, from
> its bare walls, the monotonous uniforms
> and rows of beds...

Manassein advocated the utilization of music in hospitals as well as occupational therapy and various forms of
exercise and sports events:

> Every well-organized hospital should have
> various devices for the occupation and
> amusement of patients, for example, news-
> papers, books, chess, cards, lotto,
> billiards.

He urged the institution of a program of clinical and basic
research on psychosomatic factors in therapy.

Another student of Botkin, V. P. Obraztsov (1849-1920)
(see Obraztsov, 1950) called attention to the close relationship between the disturbances of visceral and somatic
functions, problems of referred pain, the neurasthenic heart,
and the role of autosuggestion in cardiovascular disease.

It is worth mentioning that Sigmund Freud did not start
out as a proponent of Cartesian brain-mind dualism. In the
introduction to his last neurologically oriented work, The
Project (written in 1895, see Freud, 1954), Freud stated:

> The intention of this project is to
> furnish us with a psychology which
> shall be a natural science: its aim,
> that is, is to represent psychical
> processes as quantitatively determined
> states of specifiable material particles...
> the material particles in question are the
> neurons.

The hindrance constituted by the mechanistic-anatomic
approach in studying mental functions can be detected in
Freud's own revealing succinct statement made in 1915, some
two decades after the initiation of his psychoanalytic work
(Freud, 1953, p. 107):

> Research has afforded irrefutable proof
> that mental activity is bound up with the
> functions of the brain...But every attempt
> to deduce from these facts a localization
> of mental processes, every endeavor to
> think of ideas as stored up in nerve cells...
> has completely miscarried...Here there is
> a hiatus which at present can not be filled...
> Our mental topography has for the present
> nothing to do with anatomy; it is concerned
> not with anatomical locations, but with the
> regions in the mental apparatus, irrespec-
> tive of their possible position in the body.
> In this respect then our work is untrammeled
> and may proceed according to its own re-
> quirements.

It is apparent from Freud's writings that he went
through a period of agonizing intellectual inner struggles
and soul-searching before he abandoned the objective

scientific method in which he was trained in neurology in
favor of subjective introspective techniques.

Some Pavlovians claim that in developing his concepts,
Freud deliberately ignored Pavlov's contributions. But one
must recall that Freud published his book The Interpretation
of Dreams in 1900, three years before Pavlov presented his
first paper on conditioning at the International Medical
Congress in Madrid (see Pavlov, 1903, 1951) and twenty-three
years before the first publication of Pavlov's collected
papers (in Russian).

In his attempt to elucidate the nature of mental diseases,
Freud was faced with difficult philosophical, methodological,
and practical obstacles. He was trained as a neurologist,
accustomed to look for specific anatomic-histologic links to
disease processes. Such techniques obviously could not give
him the answers. In addition, Freud was faced with the practical problem of treating patients in order to earn a living.
An attempt to enter an academic career would have represented
a highly dubious undertaking even for a man as brilliant as
Freud, considering the problem of race prejudice in academic
circles at that time.

Homer Smith (1953, 1959), in describing the nature of
the scientific method, pointed out elegantly the pitfalls of
premature conclusions:

> In essence, the scientific method consists
> of careful observation of nature and cautious
> confirmation of all conclusions, to the ex-
> clusion of unsubstantiated hypotheses. A
> scientist is one who, when he does not know
> the answer, is rigorously disciplined to
> speak up and say so unashamedly; which is the
> essential feature by which modern science is
> distinguished from primitive superstition,
> which knew all the answers except how to say,
> 'I do not know.' On every scientist's desk
> there is a drawer labeled 'unknown' in which
> he files what are at the moment unsolved
> questions, lest through guesswork or impatient
> speculation he come upon incorrect answers
> that will do him more harm than good. Man's
> worst fault is opening the drawer too soon.

His task is not to discover final answers
but to win the best partial answers that
he can, from which others may move con-
fidently against the unknown, to win
better ones.

It would appear that perhaps Freud opened the "unknown" drawer prematurely; forced to do so because at the
time when he needed the answers, no other drawers with useful data were available. The criticism leveled by Pavlovians and proponents of behavioral therapy is that some of
the latter-day followers of Freud spend too much time looking in the same drawers and are not paying enough attention
to the files containing experimentally verifiable data and
concepts, and what is even more important, to files containing theoretical constructs which could be subjected to
experimental verification.

In evaluating Freud's contributions, one must view his
work in proper historical perspective. In spite of the fact
that he was tackling difficult problems before appropriate
technology became available, Freud did make some significant
contributions. Freud must be given credit for emphasizing
the importance of early postnatal experience and the role
of the subconscious and of repression in psychopathology.

There is little doubt that early postnatal experience
may modify significantly behavioral patterns in adulthood,
as has been demonstrated by Ader (1966), Fuller and Waller
(1962), Harlow (1962), Hess (1962), Levine (1962), Scott
and Fuller (1965), and Pavlov (1934, 1955).

III.   PAVLOVIAN TYPOLOGY AND CONSTITUTIONAL DIFFERENCES
       IN REACTIONS TO PSYCHOSOCIAL FACTORS

Medical and veterinary clinicians, animal breeders, and
observant farmers have long been aware of marked individual
differences in the susceptibility of living organisms to
disease, responsivity to injury and drugs, and behavioral
patterns. Yet, scientific investigations of individual
differences in the biological and behavioral sciences have
lagged far behind the massive efforts expended on studies of
average reactions.

As early as 1865, Claude Bernard cautioned biologists
against the misuse of statistical methods in describing

averages that have no relationship to biologic reality. He
quoted as an example of such a pursuit of a mythical average
the case of "a physiologist who took urine from a railroad
station urinal where people of all nations passed, and who
believed he could thus present an analysis of average
European urine!"

Just as Bernard foreshadowed the development of the
concept of biochemical and physiologic homeostasis and
cybernetics, so he was also able to discern the principles
of biologic individuality. Thus, Bernard stated:

> By destroying the biological character of
> the phenomena, the use of averages in
> physiology and medicine usually gives only
> apparent accuracy to the results...Averages
> ...confuse while aiming to unify and dis-
> tort while aiming to simplify.

Reductionist physiologists succeeded in obliterating
biologic individuality not only by the misapplication of
statistical methods but also by limiting their experiments
to anesthetized (and often macerated) animals and isolated
organs and tissues. In this manner they managed to oblit-
erate not only constitutional differences but also variations
associated with biological rhythms and environmental changes.

This is not to disparage reductionism per se or the
fractional-analytic approach in biomedical and psychobiologic
research. Such analytic studies have made, and will continue
to make, essential contributions to biological and behavioral
sciences. The argument is not for abolishing reductionist-
analytic studies. Rather, it is to assert that: a) the
functioning of biologic organisms cannot be understood by
merely studying the individual components of the living machinery and b) the mechanisms of sexual reproduction run
counter to the concept of an "average standard machinery" in
living organisms.

Hirsch (1967) epitomized the glaring neglect of individual differences in the behavioral and psychobiological sci-
sciences by the following rather pithy statement:

> The 50-year fiasco that was behaviorism,
> what the Brelands (1961) correctly called
> 'a clear and utter failure of conditioning

> theory,' resulted from a blind fixation on
> the impossible task of trying to generalize
> about 'laws' of environmental influence.

Hirsch and Tryon (1956) pointed out that

> it is patent...that environmental influ-
> ence must be an influence on something
> and therefore the laws of such influence
> must differ as the object influenced
> differs.

It was I. P. Pavlov who must be credited with initiating one of the first systematic longitudinal investigations of individual behavioral and psychophysiologic differences in dogs. As early as 1907-08, three of Pavlov's students pub-lished dissertations on individual differences exhibited by dogs in the course of elaboration of conditioned reflexes (Pimenov, 1907; Perel'tsveig, 1907; Zavadskii, 1908). These early observations were related chiefly to differences in general motor behavior on the Pavlovian stand during salivary conditioning experiments and in the dog kennels.

There has been a great deal of confusion regarding Pav-lovian typology in the Western and even the Russian literature This confusion can be ascribed to three factors: 1) Pavlov gradually evolved different conceptual constructs for typology 2) perversion of the Pavlovian typology concepts by political pressures from the Soviet brand of behaviorism generated by Lysenkoism; and 3) the word "typology" has been used by some American behavior-geneticists in a different sense from that used by the Pavlovian school. We therefore propose to review briefly the development of Pavlovian typology concepts and to relate these concepts to current studies on individual dif-ferences.

The first systematic attempt in Pavlov's laboratory to classify dogs according to their individual differences in patterns of behavior was made by Nikiforovskii (1910). He classified the dogs into three types: a) extremely excitable, nervous, sensitive dogs; b) extremely inhibitory, unexcitable dogs; and c) a central intermediate type in which he placed the majority of dogs he studied. This classification was based entirely on relatively superficial indices of the bal-ance between excitation and inhibition in general patterns of behavior in dogs during conditioning experiments.

In 1925 in a paper entitled "Normal and Pathological States of the Cerebral Hemispheres" (see Pavlov, 1954), Pavlov proposed his first typology scheme based on observations of general patterns of behavior and also on basic properties of the central nervous system as derived from studies on the development of conditional reflexes. Two properties of the central nervous system were considered: the strength of cortical cells ("the supply of excitatory substance in the cortical cells") and the balance between excitation and inhibition. He proposed four types: 1) an extreme excitatory type--strong (sanguinic); 2) an extreme inhibitory type--weak (melancholic); and two intermediate types--choleric (approximating the sanguinic) and phlegmatic (approximating the melancholic).

In 1927 in a paper entitled "Physiological Investigations on the Types of Nervous System, i.e., of Temperaments" (see Pavlov, 1954), Pavlov switched the positions of the sanguinic and choleric types. These confusing changing classifications were due to the fact that Pavlov initially used, as criteria for his typology, indices derived from investigations on the basic properties of the central nervous system, as well as from observations of the general behavior of the dogs. For example, one of the indices for classifying a dog as belonging to the "weak" type was "cowardice" (timidity) or the presence of a "passive defense reflex".

However, Vyrzhikhovskii and Maiorov (1933) and Zeval'd (1938) demonstrated that timidity does not necessarily indicate that the dog belongs to a "weak" type in terms of basic properties of the central nervous system as derived from salivary conditioning experiments. Vyrzhikhovskii and Maiorov took eight puppies from two litters and raised half of them in isolation cages for a period of two years and the other half in the usual laboratory conditions with a comparatively enriched environment. All the dogs raised in the isolation cages turned out to be timid, but none of them belonged to the "inhibitory" or "weak" type when tested in salivary conditioning experiments. It thus appeared that while early isolation may modify the general behavior of dogs, it did not seem to change significantly the basic properties of the nervous system.

For this reason, during the years 1933-36 Pavlov eliminated the consideration of general patterns of behavior from the typologic classification. From this period on, the

Pavlovian typology was based entirely on the following
criteria derived solely from salivary conditioning experiments: strength of the nervous system, balance between
excitation and inhibition, and mobility or lability of the
nervous system. This definitive classification scheme was
as follows:

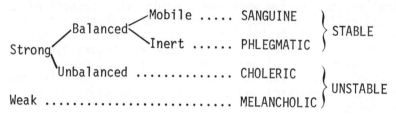

It is not feasible within the limits of this short
survey to describe the details of the methods of determining
Pavlovian typology. Briefly, the strength of the nervous
processes is estimated by determining the threshold of the
appearance of the so-called "supramaximal inhibition" (also
translated as "supramarginal" or "transmarginal") in response
to the application of progressively stronger or more prolonged stimuli or stimuli presented at higher frequencies.
The Russian phrase Pavlov used was "zapredel'noe tormozhenie",
which literally means "inhibition beyond the limit". In
physiologic terms this phrase could best be rendered as
"supraoptimal inhibition". It implies that for any individual
animal there is an optimal intensity, frequency, or duration
of stimuli that will evoke a response. Stimuli exceeding
these values will evoke inhibition. "Strong" types will exhibit a higher threshold before supraoptimal inhibition will
appear.

The balance of nervous processes is determined by the
relative ease of elaboration of positive and negative conditional reflexes, i.e., by the number of reinforcements required to produce a positive CR and the number of presenta-
tions of unreinforced differentiating stimuli required to
develop differentiation or a negative CR.

Mobility or lability is estimated by the ease of con-
version of a positive conditional reflex into a negative
conditional reflex and vice versa; e.g., in so-called
"switching" experiments, when a negative conditional stimulus
is reinforced while the previously positive conditional stimulus is not reinforced.

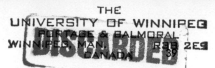
THE
UNIVERSITY OF WINNIPEG
PORTAGE & BALMORAL
WINNIPEG, MAN.   R3B 2E9
CANADA
DISCARDED

Numerous other experimental procedures have been used
for the estimation of the three basic properties of the
nervous system and the final determination of the typology.
They are all based on longitudinal conditioning experiments.
The original battery of tests devised in Pavlov's laboratories during the years 1934-41 is known as the "large
standard" and requires experiments lasting 1½ to two years.
Kolesnikov and Troshikhin (1951) introduced the so-called
"small standard" requiring only about six months.

The significant conclusions that emanate from reviewing
Pavlovian typology studies may be summarized as follows:

1. Pavlov recognized the importance of conducting
longitudinal studies (what he referred to as "chronic experiments") in discerning constitutional differences.

2. In his final formulation, after some 30 years of
experimentation, Pavlov spoke about "type of nervous system",
which he equated to the "genotype" and also to the animal's
"temperament". The pattern of general behavior of the dogs
resulting from genetic and environmental interactions, Pavlov
referred to as the "phenotype" or "character". In other
words, Pavlov concluded that, whereas the general behavior
of the animals may be significantly modified by environmental
events, the basic types of the central nervous system remain
relatively stable.

What Pavlov tried to emphasize was that the three basic
CNS properties as tested in the laboratory could not be significantly changed by modifying the environment, including
early postnatal experience. Pavlov realized the inadequacy
of their rather limited attempts to modify the early postnatal experience of the dog and also the inadequacy of their
tests to determine typology. Because of the widespread confusion on this score in the Russian and English literature,
it is worth quoting Pavlov (1935, "General Types of Higher
Nervous Activity in Animals and Man"; see Pavlov, 1954,
p. 144):

> We must emphasize one very essential and
> thus far almost insurmountable difficulty
> in the determination of the types of
> nervous activity. The pattern of human
> and animal behavior is determined not only
> by congenital properties of the nervous

DISCARDED

system, but also by those influences which
have impinged and continue to impinge on the
organism during its individual existence,
i.e., on the continuous education and training in the broad sense of these words. This
is so because, side by side with the above-
mentioned properties of the nervous system
(strength, balance, mobility or lability -
SAC), another most important characteristic
continually manifests itself - marked
plasticity. Consequently, since we are
talking about the innate type of nervous
system, we must take into account all those
influences to which a given organism has
been exposed from the day of its birth
until now. With regard to our experimental
material (dogs), thus far in the overwhelming majority of cases, this requirement remains only a fervent wish. We shall be able
to achieve this only when all our dogs will
be born and reared before our eyes under
our unremitting observation...(emphasis
SAC). For the elimination of the above
difficulty, thus far there is only one
remedy - to increase and diversify the
forms of our diagnostic tests, with the
idea that in this or that case the specific
changes in the innate type of nervous system occasioned by definite influences on
the individual existence will become manifest (emphasis SAC).

In his latest writings, Pavlov used the terms "congeni-
tal" or "innate" rather than "inherited" types because
Kupalov (cited by Teplov, 1961, p. 384) demonstrated that
the "innate" properties of the nervous system may be influenced by intrauterine development and by very early postnatal
environemtnal conditions.

In the West, as well as in the USSR, there has been some
misinterpretation of Pavlov's tentative classification by
transforming it into a rigid catechism of four types, no more
and no less. Pavlov actually estimated at least 24 possible
types (Teplov, 1961, p. 465). Krasuskii (1964), in his analysis of data on 116 dogs at the Pavlov Institute of Physiology at Koltushi, came up with 48 types.

Teplov (1961) pointed out that the typology of a given dog may vary depending on: a) the type of reinforcement used, b) the kind of conditional responses used as indices, and c) the modality of the conditional stimuli used. For example, Vatsuro (1949) reported that in dogs the auditory analyzer exhibits greater mobility than the visual analyzer. In the anthropoids, the kinesthetic analyzer exhibits greater mobility than the visual analyzer. Vatsuro referred to these observations as the "principle of leading afferentation".

The confusion regarding the principles of Pavlovian typology was compounded by the fact that in the English literature on behavior genetics the work "typology" has been used in a different sense from that used by Pavlov and his students. Whereas Pavlov in his latest formulation considered the types of nervous system in dogs as genotypes, Mayr (1958, 1959) and Hirsch (1962, 1967) used the word "typology" to describe behavioral-science research which "was pre-Mendelian, in fact pre-Darwinian" (Hirsch, 1967). Mayr (1958) described his typology concept thus:

> The philosophical basis in much of early science was typological, going back to the eidos of Plato. This implies that the 'typical' aspects of the phenomenon can be described, and that all variation is due to imperfect replicas of the type...The typological concept has been completely displaced in evolutionary biology by the population concept. The basis of this concept is that in sexually reproducing species no two individuals are genetically alike... The time has come to stress the existence of genetic differences in behavior.

Hirsch (1967) stated: "There is no place for individual differences in the typological frame (uniformity is axiomatic)."

It is unfortunate that the word "typology" came to be used in such a manner as to denote precisely opposite concepts. This again suggests the usefulness of a careful study of the classics in biology. Since Pavlov used "types of nervous system" to describe individual inborn differences in CNS functioning, it obviously would have been desirable not to use the same word to describe the behaviorist denial of

individual differences. Since Pavlovian "typology" is based
on the recognition of individual genetic differences in higher nervous activity, it does not represent "typological"
thinking as defined by behavior geneticists.

Some of the most extensive studies on individual differences were conducted by Petrova (1955) on dogs and by
Fedorov (1952) on dogs, mice, and human subjects. Krushinskii (1960) initiated behavioral studies on pure breeds of
dogs raised in a relatively enriched environment (private
homes) and in restricted laboratory kennels. He reported
that in both environments a greater proportion of German
shepherds developed timidity than Airedale terriers. When
German shepherds and Doberman pinschers were raised in isolation cages, 49% of the German shepherds developed excessive timidity, whereas only 12% of the Doberman pinschers
developed timidity, and only of a minimal kind.

Kavetskii et al (1961), at the Bogomolets Institute of
Physiology in Kiev, studied a number of visceral-autonomic
reactions of dogs with respect to Pavlovian typology. However, these workers limited their observations to the recording of one or two parameters without any attempts to
investigate patterns of adaptive reactions. Firsov (1961)
reported individual differences in some visceral reactions
of chimpanzees. Monaenkov (1963) summarized rather extensive experiments on individual differences in the development of immunity in rats, rabbits, and horses.

Probably some of the most sophisticated and best-con-
trolled studies in the USSR on individual differences in
human subjects have been conducted by Teplov (1961) and
Nebylitsyn (1966) at the Institute of Psychology in Moscow.
Teplov was one of the first Soviet psychologists to present
a critique of the perversion of the concepts of Pavlovian
typology and the canonization of a rigid scheme of four types.
Some publications from Teplov's laboratories were translated
by Gray (1964).

As pointed out earlier, systematic neglect of individual
differences fairly well characterized Western biologic and
psychologic research until recent times. Roger Williams
(1956) pioneered in investigating biochemical individual
differences.

Some of the early studies on genetics and behavior were conducted by Tolman (1924), Tryon (1929, 1940), and Heron (1935), who investigated the inheritance of maze-learning in rats. Searle (1949), a student of Tryon, pointed out that fear of the mechanical maze was partly responsible for the slow learning of the "dull" rats. Hall (1941), Broadhurst and Levine (1963), and Broadhurst and Eysenck (1965) reported on genetic differences in emotional responses of rats (defecation). Broadhurst (1960) summarized his extensive experiments in biometrical psychogenetics involving the diallele cross method on six strains of rats in which ambulation and defecation scores were recorded. Ginsburg (1967) studied genetics of audiogenic seizure susceptibility in mice. Bovet et al (1969) summarized their extensive studies on genetic aspects of learning and memory in mice.

Comparatively few studies have been conducted in the West on individual differences in dogs. Stockard et al (1941) attempted to investigate variations in the size of different endocrine glands in relation to behavior in several breeds of dogs. Unfortunately, Stockard died before these studies were completed.

Fuller and Thompson (1960) summarized the investigations in this area in their monograph on Behavior Genetics. Scott and Fuller (1965) presented a thorough and critical review of their work on Genetics and the Social Behavior of the Dog.

Parnell (1958) and Oganesyan (1961) summarized investigations relating somatotypes and behavior in human subjects. Anastasi (1954, 1958), Benjamin (1962), Kallmann (1954, 1962), and Vandenberg (1965) summarized the literature on genetic factors in psychiatric disturbances.

Eysenck (1960, 1963) attempted to relate Pavlov's concepts on the interaction of excitation and inhibition to extroversion and introversion in human subjects. Eysenck postulates that extroverts are characterized by a high and relatively persistent cortical inhibition, whereas introverts are characterized by a low level of cortical inhibition. When Eysenck speaks of a high degree of cortical inhibition he does not use this term in the same sense in which it is commonly used, i.e., inhibition exerted by the cortex on subcortical structures. Rather, Eysenck uses this expression to signify that the inhibited cortex has a low excitability

and therefore <u>does not inhibit the subcortical structures</u>
and thus leads to uninhibited behavior. He further reasons
that because of the low cortical inhibition (i.e., high
cortical excitation) "introverts should condition better
than extroverts." Using eyeblink conditioning tests, Eysenck
reports that this is indeed so. He then goes on to say that
since

> phobias, anxieties, obsessional and com-
> pulsive behavior patterns, etc. are nothing
> more than conditioned autonomic and skele-
> tal responses...such conditioned responses
> are more likely to occur in individuals
> predisposed to the development of conditioned
> responses by the possession of a central
> nervous system which conditions easily.
> Thus we would expect...that neurotics of this
> type would be introverts...and would also
> condition extremely well. There is much
> impressive evidence to support both these
> deductions.

Few systematic studies have been conducted with regard
to physiologic, endocrine, and biochemical mechanisms underlying individual differences in responses to psychologic
stress. Levine and Treiman (1964) reported significant
differences in the temporal patterns of plasma corticosterone
responses to noxious stimuli or novel situations in four
inbred strains of mice. Hamburg (1967), in an erudite review on "Genetics of Adrenocortical Hormone Metabolism in
Relation to Psychological Stress", reported evidence on
"genetically determined enzymatic differences in the synthesis or disposal of adrenocortical hormones." He also
reported unpublished observations by Mason and Hamburg on
"individual differences (in human subjects) in 17-hydroxy-
corticosteroid excretion, consistent over several months and
through several stressful experiences." Mason (1968), in a
thought-provoking review of his extensive concurrent measurements of endocrine responses in 72-hour avoidance session
in monkeys, called attention to significant individual differences. He concluded that

> the individual difference phenomenon is
> emerging as a central problem in psycho-
> endocrine research and the need for long-
> term systematic investigations in this
> area...seems increasingly evident.

Our own studies on mongrel and several pure breed dogs demonstrated persistent marked constitutional differences in endocrine, renal, cardiac, and respiratory reactions associated with the development of Pavlovian conditional motor defense reflexes (Corson, 1971; Corson and Corson, 1971).

Apart from the confusion regarding Pavlovian typology, Pavlovian psychobiology is often being confounded in the West with mechanistic reductionist behaviorism. It is curious that in reviewing extensively the background for the development of organismic biology, von Bertalanffy (1969) failed to mention Sechenov or Botkin and referred to Pavlov's contributions as furnishing support for the mechanistic approach in biology. This is precisely where the Sechenov-Botkin-Pavlov school does not belong.

Pavlov's significant contributions to integrative psychobiology may be summarized as follows:

1. The recognition that living organisms are goal-directed self-regulating systems. Pavlov referred to this as the "reflex of purpose or goal reflex" (Pavlov, 1916).

2. The development of techniques for psychophysiologic studies of intact unanesthetized animals.

3. The recognition of psychophysiologic constitutional differences (Pavlovian typology).

4. The emphasis on the need for longitudinal chronic studies in psychophysiologic investigations.

5. The recognition of specific human psychophysiologic characteristics and the delineation of the importance of the second signal system (language).

Pavlov's recognition of the importance of symbolic and cultural factors in human behavior can be seen from his remarks in his paper on the Reflex of Purpose (Pavlov, 1916, 1951):

> The Reflex of Purpose (goal reflex) has great vital significance; it represents the basic form of vital energy in everyone of us...all of life, all its improvements, all its culture is achieved through the reflex

of purpose, is achieved only by those
individuals who strive to reach this or
that life goal which they placed before
themselves...In contrast, life ceases
to be attractive as soon as the purpose
disappears. Do we not often read in the
notes left by suicide victims that they
ended their life because it was purpose-
less.

It is impossible within the confines of this introductory article to encompass the broad sweep of Pavlovian psychobiology. In closing one should mention the achievements of
one of Pavlov's most brilliant and imaginative students,
Peter Kuz'mich Anokhin. Having studied with Vladimir
Bekhterev (at the Brain Research Institute) before coming to
Pavlov's laboratory, Anokhin attempted to achieve a synthesis
of Pavlov's basic conditioning studies with Bekhterev's keen
clinical psychiatric and neurologic observations and his
pioneering studies on behavior modification and group psychotherapy methods.

Anokhin was one of the first in the USSR to initiate
systematic utilizations of electrophysiologic techniques in
the investigation of conditional reflexes and their role in
biological adaptation.

Anokhin also had the unique distinction of initiating a
systematic dialogue and synthesis between the Pavlovian
school and Western neurophysiology, experimental psychology,
and cybernetics. As early as 1935, Anokhin published a paper
in which he developed the concept of the functional system
as the basic unit of neurophysiologic integration, incorporating into this concept the notion of "return afferentation",
thus foreshadowing the development of the concepts of feedback, and a systems approach in psychobiology long before the
publication of Wiener's Cybernetics in 1948. Anokhin's extensive studies and original concepts are elegantly summarized in an expanded English translation of his latest book
(Anokhin, 1974).

Another important development in Pavlovian psychobiology
includes studies on the psychophysiologic basis of psychosomatic medicine, referred to by Soviet scientists as corticovisceral physiology and pathophysiology or corticovisceral

medicine. These investigations have been conducted chiefly
by Bykov and Kurtsin (1960, 1966). An extensive critical
review of this area has recently been published by Corson
and Corson (1975).

BIBLIOGRAPHY

ADER, ROBERT (1966). Early experience and adaptation to
    stress. Res. Publ. Ass. Nerv. Ment. Dis., Williams
    & Wilkins, Baltimore, 43:292-308.

ANASTASI, ANNE (1954). The inherited and acquired compon-
    ents of behavior. In: Genetics and the Inheritance
    of Integrated Neurological and Psychiatric Patterns.
    Davenport Hooker and Clarence C. Hare, eds. Williams
    & Wilkins Co., Baltimore, pp. 67-75.

ANASTASI, ANNE (1958). Heredity, environment, and the
    question,"How?". Psychol. Rev. 65:197-208.

ANOKHIN, P. K. (1935). Problema tsentra i periferii v
    sovremennoi fiziologii nervnoi deyatel'nosti (The
    problem of center and periphery in modern physiology
    of nervous activity). In: Problema tsentra i periferii
    v fiziologii nervnoi deyatel'nosti (The Problem of Center
    and Periphery in the Physiology of Nervous Activity),
    P. K. Anokhin, ed. Gosizdat, Gorki, pp. 1-70.

ANOKHIN, P. K. (1962). Refleks tseli, kak ob"ekt fiziologi-
    cheskogo analiza (The reflex of purpose as the object
    of physiologic analysis). Zh. vyssh. nervn. deyat. im.
    I. P. Pavlova (I. P. Pavlov Journal of Higher Nervous
    Activity) 12(1):7-21.

ANOKHIN, P. K. (1974). Biology and Neurophysiology of the
    Conditioned Reflex and Its Role in Adaptive Behavior,
    Samuel A. Corson, Scientific and Translation Editor.
    International Series of Monographs on Cerebrovisceral
    and Behavioral Physiology and Conditioned Reflexes,
    Volume 3. Pergamon Press, Oxford and New York, 574 pp.
    Translation of Biologiya i neirofiziologiya uslovnogo
    refleksa (1968).

BENJAMIN, JOHN D. (1962). Some comments on twin research
    in psychiatry. In: Research Approaches to Psychiatric
    Problems, T. T. Tourlentes, S. L. Pollack, and H. E.
    Himwich, eds. Grune and Stratton, New York, pp. 92-112.

BERNARD, CLAUDE (1859). Leçons sur les propriétés physiol-
    ogiques et les altérations pathologiques des liquides
    de l'organisme (Lessons on the Physiological Properties
    and the Pathological Changes of the Body Fluids). Paris.

BERNARD, CLAUDE (1865). Introduction à l'étude de la mé-
    decine expérimentale. Paris. English edition: An
    Introduction to the Study of Experimental Medicine.
    Dover Publications, New York, 1957.

BERTALANFFY, LUDWIG VON (1969). General System Theory.
    Foundations, Development, Applications. Braziller,
    New York, xvi, 290 pp.

BOVET, D., F. BOVET-NITTI, and A. OLIVERIO (1969). Genetic
    aspects of learning and memory in mice. Science
    163:139-149.

BRAZIER, MARY A. B. (1959). The historical development of
    neurophysiology. Handbook of Physiology, Section 1,
    1:1-58, Amer. Physiol. Society, Washington, D. C.

BRELAND, K. and M. BRELAND (1961). The misbehavior of or-
    ganisms. Amer. Psychol. 16:681-684.

BROADHURST, P. L. (1960). Applications of biometrical gene-
    tics to the inheritance of behaviour. In: Experiments
    in Personality. H. J. Eysenck, ed. Humanities Press,
    New York.

BROADHURST, P. L. and H. J. EYSENCK (1965). Emotionality
    in the rat: a problem of response specificity. In:
    Stephanos: Studies in Psychology Presented to Cyril
    Burt. C. Banks and P. L. Broadhurst, eds. pp. 205-222

BROADHURST, P. L. and S. LEVINE (1963). Behavioral consis-
    tency in strains of rats selectively bred for emotional
    elimination. Brit. J. Psychol. 54:121-125.

BYKOV, K. M., and I. T. KURTSIN (1960). Kortiko-vistseral'-naya patologiya (Corticovisceral Pathology). Medgiz, Leningrad, 576 pp. A revised English edition has been prepared by Samuel A. Corson.

BYKOV, K. M. and I. T. KURTSIN (1966). The Corticovisceral Theory of the Pathogenesis of Peptic Ulcer, Samuel A. Corson, Scientific and Translation Editor. International Series of Monographs on Cerebrovisceral and Behavioural Physiology and Conditioned Reflexes, Volume 2. Pergamon Press, London, 1966. Translation of Kortiko-vistseral'naya teoriya patogeneza yazvennoi bolezni, 1952.

CANNON, WALTER B. (1929). Bodily Changes In Pain, Hunger, Fear, and Rage. 2nd Edition, Appleton, New York.

CANNON, WALTER B. (1932). The Wisdom of the Body. W. W. Norton and Company, New York.

CHERNYSHEVSKII, N. G. (1860). Antropologicheskii printsip v filosofii (The Anthropologic Principle in Philosophy). Reprinted: Moscow, 1948.

CORSON, SAMUEL A. (1957). Review of: F. R. Borodulin. S. P. Botkin and the Neurogenic Theory of Medicine. Medgiz, Moscow, 2nd edition, 1953. 184 pp. (In Russian). Science 125(3237):75-77, 1957.

CORSON, SAMUEL A. (1971). Pavlovian and operant conditioning techniques in the study of psychosocial and biological relationships. In: Society, Stress and Disease. Volume 1. The Psychosocial Environment and Psychosomatic Diseases, Lennart Levi, ed. Oxford University Press, London, pp. 7-21.

CORSON, SAMUEL A. and ELIZABETH O'LEARY CORSON (1971). Psychosocial influences on renal function - implications for human pathophysiology. In: Society, Stress and Disease. Volume 1. The Psychosocial Environment and Psychosomatic Diseases, Lennart Levi, ed. Oxford University Press, London, pp. 338-351.

CORSON, SAMUEL A. and E. O'LEARY CORSON (1975). Cerebrovisceral physiology and pathophysiology and psychosomatic
medicine. Totus Homo 6(1-3):85-123.

EYSENCK, H. J., ed. (1960). Experiments in Personality.
Volume 1: Psychogenetics and psychopharmacology.
Humanities Press, Inc., New York.

EYSENCK, H. J. (1963). Biological basis of personality.
Nature 199(4898):1031-1034.

FEDOROV, V. K. (1952). Znachenie dlya psikhiatrii i psikho-
logii ucheniya I. P. Pavlova o tipakh vysshei nervnoi
deyatel'nosti. (Significance of I. P. Pavlov's teaching on types of higher nervous activity for psychiatry
and psychology). Zh. Nevropatol. i Psikhiat. 52(6):
13-19.

FIRSOV, L. A. (1961). Sravnitel'naya kharakteristika
povedeniya i nekotorykh vegetativnykh funktsii u
shimpanze (Comparative characteristics of behavior
and of some vegetative functions in the chimpanzee).
Dokl. Akad. nauk SSSR 141(6):1522-1524.

FREUD, SIGMUND (1953). Collected Papers. Volume IV.
Hogarth Press, London, p. 107.

FREUD, SIGMUND (1954). The Origin of Psychoanalysis.
New York, 255 pp.

FULLER, J. L. and W. R. THOMPSON (1960). Behavior Genetics.
John Wiley and Sons, New York-London-Sydney.

FULLER, JOHN L. and MARCUS B. WALLER (1962). Is early
experience different? In: Roots of Behavior, Eugene
L. Bliss, ed. Harper and Brothers, New York, pp. 235-
245.

FULTON, JOHN F. (1949 a). Functional Localization in Relation to Frontal Lobotomy. Oxford University Press,
New York-London, 140 pp.

FULTON, JOHN F. (1949 b). Physiology of the Nervous System.
Oxford University Press, New York, Third Edition, x,
667 pp.

GANTT, W. HORSLEY (1944). Experimental Basis for Neurotic
Behavior. Hoeber, New York, 211 pp.

GANTT, W. HORSLEY (1953). Principles of nervous breakdown -
schizokinesis and autokinesis. Ann. N. Y. Acad. Sci.
56(2):143-163.

GANTT, W. HORSLEY (1960). Cardiovascular component of the
conditional reflex to pain, food and other stimuli.
Physiol. Rev. 40(Suppl. 4):266-291.

GANTT, W. HORSLEY (1962). Factors involved in the development of pathological behavior: schizokinesis and autokinesis. Perspectives Biol. Med. 5(4):473-482.

GINETSINSKII, A. G. (1963). Fiziologicheskie mekhanizmy
vodno-solevogo ravnovesiya. (The Physiologic Mechanisms of Water-Salt Balance). Akademiya Nauk SSSR,
Moscow - Leningrad, 428 pp.

GINSBURG, BENSON E. (1967). Genetic parameters in behavioral
research. In: Behavior-Genetic Analysis, J. Hirsch, ed.
McGraw-Hill, New York.

GRAY, J. A., ed. (1964). Pavlov's Typology. Pergamon Press,
Oxford-New York.

HALL, C. S. (1941). Temperament: a survey of animal studies.
Psychol. Bull. 38:909-943.

HAMBURG, DAVID A. (1967). Genetics of adrenocortical hor-
mone metabolism in relation to psychological stress.
In: Behavior-Genetic Analysis, J. Hirsch, ed. McGraw-
Hill, New York.

HAMBURG, DAVID A. (1971). Crowding, stranger contact, and
aggressive behaviour. In: Society, Stress and Disease.
Volume 1. The Psychosocial Environment and Psychosomatic Diseases, Lennart Levi, ed. Oxford University Press,
London, pp. 209-218.

HARLOW, HARRY F. (1962). Development of affection in primates. In: Roots of Behavior, Eugene L. Bliss, ed.
Harper and Brothers, New York, pp. 157-166.

HERON, W. T. (1935). The inheritance of maze-learning
     ability in rats. J. Comp. Psychol. 19:77-89.

HESS, ECKHARD H. (1962). Imprinting and the "critical
     period" concept. In: Roots of Behavior, Eugene
     L. Bliss, ed. Harper and Brothers, New York, pp.
     254-263.

HIRSCH, J. (1962). Individual differences in behavior and
     their genetic basis. In: Roots of Behavior, Eugene
     L. Bliss, ed. Harper and Brothers, New York, pp. 3-23.

HIRSCH, J. (1967). Behavior-genetic analysis. In: Behav-
     ior-Genetic Analysis, J. Hirsch, ed. McGraw-Hill, New
     York, pp. 416-435.

HIRSCH, J. and R. C. TRYON (1956). Mass screening and re-
     liable individual measurements in the experimental be-
     havior genetics of lower organisms. Psychol. Bull.
     53:402-410.

KALLMANN, FRANZ J. (1954). The genetics of psychotic be-
     havior patterns. In: Genetics and the Inheritance
     of Integrated Neurological and Psychiatric Patterns,
     Davenport Hooker and Clarence C. Hare, eds. Williams
     and Wilkins Co., Baltimore, pp. 357-366.

KALLMANN, FRANZ J. (1962). New genetic approaches to psy-
     chiatric disorders. In: Research Approaches to Psy-
     chiatric Problems, T. T. Tourlentes, L. Pollack, and
     H. E. Himwich, eds. Grune and Stratton, New York, pp.
     74-89.

KAVETSKII, R. E., N. F. SOLODYUK, S. I. VOVK, M. S.
     KRASNOVSKAYA, and T. A. DZGOEVA (1961). Reaktivnost'
     organizma i tip nervnoi sistemy (Reactivity of the
     Organism and Type of Nervous System). Akademiya Nauk
     USSR, Institut Fiziologii im. A. A. Bogomol'tsa, Kiev,
     328 pp.

KOLESNIKOV, M. S. and V. A. TROSHIKHIN (1951). Malyi
     standart ispytanii dlya opredeleniya tipa vysshei
     nervnoi deyatel'nosti sobaki (The small standard of
     tests for the determination of the type of higher
     nervous activity in dogs). Zh. vyssh. nerv. deyat.
     I. P. Pavlova 1(5):739-743.

KOSHTOYANTS, KH. S. (1946). Ocherki po istorii fiziologii v Rossii (Essays on the History of Physiology in Russia). Akademiya Nauk SSSR (Academy of Sciences of the USSR), Moscow, 494 pp.

KRASUSKII, V. K. (1964). Metodika otsenki svoistv nervnykh protsessov u sobak, prinyataya laboratoriei fiziologii i genetiki tipov vysshei nervnoi deyatel'nosti. (The method of evaluation of the properties of nervous processes in dogs adopted by the laboratory of the physiology and genetics of types of higher nervous activity). In: Chernigovskii, V. N. Metodiki izucheniya tipologicheskikh osobennostei vysshei nervnoi deyatel'nosti zhivotnykh (Methods of Studying the Typologic Characteristics of Higher Nervous Activity in Animals). AN SSSR, Moscow-Leningrad, 1964, pp. 197-213.

KRUSHINSKII, L. V. (1960). Formirovanie povedeniya zhivotnykh v norme i patologii (The Formation of Animal Behavior under Normal and Pathologic Conditions). Moscow University, Moscow.

LEVINE, SEYMOUR (1962). Psychophysiological effects of infantile stimulation. In: Roots of Behavior, Eugene L. Bliss, ed. Harper and Brothers, New York, pp. 246-253.

LEVINE, S. and D. M. TREIMAN (1964). Differential plasma corticosterone response to stress in four inbred strains of mice. Endocrinology 75:142-144.

LISITSYN, YU. (1961). Nervizm (Nervism). In: Bol'shaya Meditsinskaya Entsiklopediya (Large Medical Encyclopedia), A. N. Bakulev, ed. Volume 20, columns 503-510. Gosudarstvennoe Nauchnoe Izdatel'stvo "Sovetskaya Entsiklopediya", Moscow.

MANASSEIN, V. A. (1876). Materialy dlya voprosa ob etiologicheskom i terapevticheskom znachenii psikhicheskikh vliyanii (Material on the problem of the etiologic and therapeutic importance of psychic influences). St. Petersburg.

MASON, JOHN W. (1968). Organization of the multiple endocrine responses to avoidance in the monkey. Psychosom. Med. 30(5)Part 2:774-790.

MAYR, E. (1958). Behavior and systematics. In: Behavior
    and Evolution, A. Roe and G. G. Simpson, eds. Yale
    University Press, New Haven.

MAYR, E. (1959). Darwin and the evolutionary theory in
    biology. In: Evolution and Anthropology: A Centen-
    nial Appraisal, B. J. Megges, ed. The Anthropology
    Society of Washington, Washington, D. C., pp. 1-10.

MONAENKOV, A. M. (1963). Faktor individual'nosti v prots-
    essakh immuniteta (The Factor of Individuality in
    Immune Processes). Institut normal'noi i patologi-
    cheskoi fiziologii, Akademiya Meditsinskikh Nauk SSSR,
    Moscow.

NEBYLITSYN, V. D. (1966). Osnovnye svoistva nervnoi sis-
    temy cheloveka (Fundamental Properties of the Human
    Nervous System). Prosveshchenie, Moscow.

NIKIFOROVSKII, P. M. (1910). Farmakologiya uslovnykh
    refleksov, kak metod dlya ikh izucheniya. (Pharmacolo-
    gy of Conditioned Reflexes as a Method for Their Inves-
    tigation). Dissertation, St. Petersburg, 200 pp.

OBRAZTSOV, V. P. (1950). Izbrannye Trudy (Selected Papers).
    Kiev.

OGANESYAN, L. A. (1961). O vzaimootnosheniyakh mezhdu
    psikhicheskoi i somaticheskoi sferami v klinike vnu-
    trennikh boleznei (Interrelations Between the Psychic
    and Somatic Spheres in the Clinical Course of Internal
    Diseases). Institut Kardiologii, Akademiya Nauk
    Armyanskoi SSR, Erevan.

PARNELL, R. W. (1958). Behaviour and Physique. An intro-
    duction to practical and applied somatometry. Edward
    Arnold Ltd., London.

PAVLOV, I. P. (1903). Eksperimental'naya psikhologiya i
    psikhopatologiya na zhivotnykh (Experimental psycho-
    logy and psychopathology on animals). Izv. Voenno-med.
    Akad. (Bulletin of the Military Medical Academy) 7(2):
    109-121. In: Pavlov, I. P. Dvadtsatiletnii opyt ob"-
    ektivnogo izucheniya vysshei nervnoi deyatel'nosti
    (povedeniya) zhivotnykh. Uslovnye refleksy (Twenty
    Years of Experience in the Objective Study of the

Higher Nervous Activity [Behavior] of Animals. Conditioned Reflexes). Medgiz, Moscow, 1951, Chapter 1, pp. 13-23.

PAVLOV, I. P. (1916). Refleks tseli (The Reflex of Purpose). Ibid., 1951, Chapter 27, pp. 197-201.

PAVLOV, I. P. (1930). A brief outline of the higher nervous activity. In: Psychologies of 1930. Clark University Press, Worcester, Mass. Ibid., 1951, Chapter 45, pp. 313-324. Kratkii ocherk vysshei nervnoi deyatel'nosti.

PAVLOV, I. P. (1933). O vozmozhnosti slitiya sub"ektivnogo s ob"ektivnym (The Possibility of the Amalgamation of the Subjective with the Objective). Ibid., 1951, Chapter 49, p. 342.

PAVLOV, I. P. (1934). 2. Isteriya (Hysteria). Wednesday, December 5, 1934. In: Pavlovskie klinicheskie sredy (Pavlov's Clinical Wednesdays). Akademiya Nauk SSSR, Moscow-Leningrad, 1955, Volume 2, p. 296.

PAVLOV, I. P. (1935). Obshchie tipy vysshei nervnoi deyatel'nosti zhivotnykh i cheloveka (General types of higher nervous activity in animals and man). In: Poslednie soobshcheniya po fiziologii i patologii vysshei nervnoi deyatel'nosti (Latest Reports on the Physiology and Pathology of Higher Nervous Activity). Akademiya Nauk SSSR, Moscow, No. 3, pp. 5-41. Also in: Pavlov, I. P. (1954). O tipakh vysshei nervnoi deyatel'nosti i eksperimental'nykh nevrozakh (Types of Higher Nervous Activity and Experimental Neuroses), P.S. Kupalov, ed. Medgiz, Moscow, pp. 143-159.

PAVLOV, I. P. (1928). Lectures on Conditioned Reflexes, W. Horsley Gantt, translator and editor. International Publishers Co., Inc., New York (Fifth printing, 1963), 414 pp.

PAVLOV, I. P. (1941). Lectures on Conditioned Reflexes. Volume 2. Conditioned Reflexes and Psychiatry, W. Horsley Gantt, translator and editor. International Publishers Co., Inc., New York (Third printing, 1963), 199 pp.

PAVLOV, I. P. (1954). O tipakh vysshei nervnoi deyatel'-nosti i eksperimental'nykh nevrozakh (Types of Higher Nervous Activity and Experimental Neuroses). P. S. Kupalov, ed. Medgiz, Moscow, 192 pp.

PEREL'TSVEIG (PERELZVEIG), I. YA. (1907). Materialy k ucheniyu ob uslovnykh refleksakh (Materials on the Theory of Conditioned Reflexes). Dissertation, St. Petersburg, 166 pp.

PETROVA, M. K. (1955). O roli funktsional'no oslablennoi kory golovnogo mozga v vozniknovenii razlichnykh pato-logicheskikh protsessov v organizme (The Role of a Functionally Weakened Cerebral Cortex in the Onset of Various Pathologic Processes in the Organism). Medgiz, Moscow.

PIMENOV, P. P. (1907). Osobaya gruppa uslovnykh refleksov (A Particular Group of Conditional Reflexes). Disser-tation, St. Petersburg, 88 pp.

SCOTT, JOHN PAUL, and JOHN L. FULLER (1965). Genetics and the Social Behavior of the Dog. University of Chicago Press, Chicago, 468 pp.

SEARLE, L. V. (1949). The organization of hereditary maze-brightness and maze-dullness. Genet. Psychol. Mono-graph 39:279-325.

SECHENOV, I. M. (1861). Dve zaklyuchitel'nye lektsii o znachenii tak nazyvaemykh rastitel'nykh aktov v zhivo-tnoi zhizni (Two concluding lectures on the signifi-cance of the so-called vegetative functions in animal life). Med. vestn. (Medical Bulletin) No. 26:235-242 and No. 28:253-258.

SECHENOV, I. M. (1863). Refleksy golovnogo mozgo (Reflex-es of the brain). Med. vestn. (Medical Herald) No. 47:461-481 and No. 48:493-512. English edition in: I. Sechenov. Selected Physiological and Psychological Works. Foreign Languages Publishing House, Moscow, 1956, pp. 31-139.

SHERRINGTON, CHARLES S. (1941). Man on His Nature. Cam-bridge University Press, Cambridge, 413 pp. (Double-day, New York, 1953).

SHIDLOVSKII, V. (1957). Claude Bernard. In: Bol'shaya Meditsinskaya Entsiklopediya (Large Medical Encyclopedia). Sovetskaya Entsiklopediya, Moscow, Volume 3, pp. 818-821.

SMITH, HOMER W. (1953). From Fish to Philosopher. Little, Brown and Co., Boston, 264 pp. Ciba edition, revised and enlarged, 1959.

STOCKARD, CHARLES R., O. D. ANDERSON and W. T. JAMES (1941). The genetic and endocrinic basis for differences in form and behavior. In: American Anatomical Memoirs, No. 19, Wistar Inst. of Anatomy and Biology, Philadelphia.

TEPLOV, B. M. (1961). Problemy individual'nykh razlichii (Problems of Individual Differences). Akademiya Pedagogicheskikh Nauk RSFSR, Moscow.

TOLMAN, E. C. (1924). The inheritance of maze-learning ability in rats. J. Comp. Psychol. 4:1-18.

TRYON, R. C. (1929). The genetics of learning ability in rats. Univ. Calif. Publ. Psychol. 4:71-89.

TRYON, R. C. (1940). Genetic differences in maze-learning ability in rats. In: Yearbook National Soc. Stud. Educ. 39(1):111-119.

VANDENBERG, S. G. ed. (1965). Methods and Goals in Human Behavior Genetics. Academic Press, New York.

VATSURO, E. G. (1949). Printsip vedushchei afferentatsii v uchenii vysshei nervnoi deyatel'nosti (The principle of leading afferentation in the study of higher nervous activity). Fiziol. zh. SSSR 35(5).

VIRCHOW, RUDOLF (1858). Die Cellularpathologie.

VIRCHOW, RUDOLF (1958). Disease, Life and Man, Selected Essays. Translated by Helfand Rather, Stanford University Press, Stanford, California.

VYRZHIKOVSKII, S. N. and F. P. MAIOROV (1933). K voprosu o
    vliyanii vospitaniya na sklad vysshei nervnoi deyatel'-
    nosti u sobak (The influence of rearing on the consti-
    tution of higher nervous activity in dogs). Tr.
    fiziol. lab. I. P. Pavlova 5:169-191.

WIENER, NORBERT (1948). Cybernetics. John Wiley and Sons,
    New York.

WILLIAMS, ROGER J. (1956). Biochemical Individuality.
    John Wiley and Sons, New York.

ZAVADSKII, I. V. (1908). Materialy k voprosu o tormozhenii
    i rastormazhivanii uslovnykh refleksov (Inhibition and
    Disinhibition of Conditional Reflexes). Dissertation,
    St. Petersburg, 195 pp.

ZEVAL'D, L. O. (1938). K voprosu o vliyanii uslovii
    vospitaniya na sklad vysshei nervnoi deyatel'nosti
    u sobak (The influence of the conditions of rearing
    on the constitution of higher nervous activity in
    dogs). Tr. fiziol. lab. I. P. Pavlova, Volume 8.

ACKNOWLEDGMENT

     We wish to express our appreciation to Judith Smiley
and Sandra Stein for their typing of the manuscript and to
Roland Dartau for his meticulous checking of the bibliography and proofreading of the manuscript.

HISTORY OF SOVIET PSYCHOLOGY:

RECENT SOURCES OF INFORMATION IN ENGLISH (1965-1975)

Josef Brožek

Lehigh University

Bethlehem, Pennsylvania

INTRODUCTION

This "bibliography with comment" is a complement of an extensive review of Russian works on the history of psychology published in the 1960s (Brožek, 1972, 1973, 1973a, 1974, 1974a). A separate report on the current Soviet historiography of physiology and psychology covered the activities in institutes of history of science and medicine, research institutes of physiology and psychology, and university departments (Brožek, 1971). Reference was made also to the relevant museums and archives. For a bibliography of older historical writings by both Western and Soviet authors see Brožek (1968).

Mecacci's Soviet Psychology in the Western Countries (1971) provides an extensive bibliography of publications in English (as well as in German, French, and Italian): books and articles on Soviet psychology, works concerning specific scientists, anthologies and collections of papers, and articles and books by Soviet authors. The bibliography is preceded by commentary on the response of the West to the Russian (pre-1917) and Soviet work, and on the characteristics of Soviet psychology.

In the present survey the works of Western and of Soviet writers were grouped together in Part 1 and Part 2, respectively. At times such a separation does not work out well, for instance when both a Western and a Soviet author contribute an account of Soviet psychology to the same encyclopedia (Brožek, 1972; Luria, 1972).

PART I. WESTERN AUTHORS

Major Features and Events

On the pages of the journal American Psychologist comments were made on the second meeting of the Soviet Psychological Society (Brožek, 1965; cf. also Brožek, 1966) and the Society's organizational structure (Brožek, 1967); the relative strength of different research areas of Soviet psychology (Brožek, 1969); the 1968 provision for awarding advanced degrees in the area of "psychological sciences" (psikhologicheskie nauki; Brožek, 1970); and the decision of the USSR Academy of Sciences, announced in December 1971, to form in Moscow a major Institute of Psychology, with B.F. Lomov as the director (Brožek and Mecacci, 1974).

A List of Soviet Articles on Historiography of Psychology

The principal medium of publication of the Soviet contributions on historical themes is the journal Voprosy psikholog (Problems of Psychology). The 120-odd articles appearing in the journal, since its inception in 1955, were listed by Slobin (1968) with titles given in the original and in English translation.

Tabulation of this material yields an interesting "topometry" of Soviet historiography of psychology. Sixty-eight of the articles are concerned with the life and work of individuals in Russia and the USSR (over one half of the entries). Fourteen entries deal with various aspects of Soviet psychology (Soviet republics, institutions of learning, cities, Soviet psychology as a whole), 10 with various fields of Soviet psychology, 7 with theories, 3 with methods. Four address themselves to issues in historiography. Eleven entries are concerned with non-Soviet contributors to psychology and with developments abroad.

Book Lists

The lists of "Recent Russian Books in Psychology," published from time to time in the American journal Contemporary Psychology, contain a section on history (cf. Brožek and Herz, 1974). Combined, these lists provide the most complete bibliography, available in the West, of Soviet

publications on the history of psychology and the closely
related areas.

The historical publications that are listed consist,
typically, of proceedings of commemorative conferences,
memoirs, reissues of important older works (with added
historical materials), and an occasional monograph.

Book Reviews

The books published in Russian continue to be inacces-
sible, linguistically, to a large majority of Western readers.
This places special demands and significance on book reviews.
A list of book reviews, in English, was included in the
1966 Handbook of Soviet Psychology (Brožek, Hoskovec and
Slobin, 1966, pp.98-99). Here we shall note only reviews of
books directly relevant to the history of Soviet psychology,
few in number.

The author reviewed Yaroshevskii's 1966 History of
Psychology and A.V. Petrovskii's 1967 History of Soviet
Psychology (Brožek, 1969), and a collaborative work dealing
with the development of biology (Brožek, 1969a).

The All-Union Conference on Philosophical Problems of
the Physiology of Higher Nervous Activity and Psychology,
held in Moscow in 1962, was a milestone in the development of
Soviet psychology, especially in relation to the physiology
of behavior. Rahmani provided an informative review of the
proceedings (1965).

A review (Brožek, 1975) of T. Kussmann's Soviet Psychology:
Search for an Approach (1974, in German) considers at some
length the conflict between the traditional "Pavlovian" and
the "Vygotskian" interpretation of man's mental functions.
The latter stresses that man's mind is the product of his own
activity in the given socio-cultural and material environment.

Soviet Pavloviana in Review

Three valuable recent contributions (1967-1968) to our
knowledge of Pavlov's life and work were considered in an
essay review (Brožek, 1971a): 1) A volume of brief comments
and recollections, mostly published but some prepared specifically for this publication, 2) A collection of short biographies, with pictures and selective bibliographies, of

individuals who had worked with Pavlov, and 3) An outline of
the history of the I. P. Pavlov Institute of Physiology
in Leningrad.

Recent additions to the history of Soviet physiology
include two volumes on conditioned reflexes and a volume
on vision, forming a part of the new Handbook of Physiology
(in Russian); the first part of the chronicle of Pavlov's
life and work; and Pavlov's correspondence (Brožek, 1973a).

A 1966 Guide to the Perplexed

In the Spring of 1966, the Handbook of Soviet Psychology
(Slobin, 1966) was published as a special issue of the
journal Soviet Psychology and Psychiatry, to serve as a
guide for the participants in the 18th International Congress
of Psychology held in Moscow in August, 1966. The Handbook
contains a glossary (Bowden and Cole, 1966), a systematic
review of recent Soviet work (Brožek and Hoskovec, 1966),
a listing of materials in English on Soviet psychology (Brožek
Hoskovec and Slobin, 1966) and of translations (Brožek and
Hoskovec, 1966a). Elsewhere, books being translated or
to be translated were noted (Brožek and Hoskovec, 1966b).
The Handbook contains also pictures and biographies of outstanding Russian an Soviet psychologists and physiologists
(Anon., 1966). Directories of Soviet institutions (Slobin,
1966a) and of Soviet scientists active in the area of psychology and physiology (Slobin and Gordon, 1966) were added
for good measure.

O'Connor's 1966 Symposium

Following a preamble dealing with the "philosophical
roots" of Soviet psychology, Gray (1966) focuses his attention on the orienting reflex, the function and nature of
consciousness, and the mechanisms of voluntary control of
behavior (cf. Lynn, 1966a). Other contributions deal with
psychotherapy (Kirman, 1966); the use of 'cybernetic' models
in the study of perceptual-motor skills, memory, and perceptual discrimination, including the perception of speech
(Rabbitt, 1966); abnormal psychology (Lynn, 1966); psycholinguistics (Slobin, 1966); and child development (Rahmani
1966). An analysis of the 1963 Soviet literary output in
psychology and of the proceedings of the 1963 meeting of the
Soviet Society of Psychologists was presented by Brožek
(1966).

Chapters in Textbooks of the History of Psychology

References to the Russian work are made, typically, in connection with behaviorism (e.g., R. I. Watson, 1968, pp. 407-413). Watson returns to the topic, briefly, in the chapter "Psychology until 1945" (pp. 518-519). A similar pattern is followed by Schultz (1975), with whom I have a bone to pick. In a comment on the developments of psychology in the Soviet Union (pp. 368-369) he notes that in the last twenty years or so "Soviet psychology has become much more active and productive. " This is true. However, this has been a consequence of de-Stalinization, not of the "Pavlovization" of Soviet psychology. The author states, incorrectly: "A turning point in the history of Soviet psychology occurred in 1950, when Pavlovian theory was given the sanction of official state doctrine" (l.c., p. 369).

Full chapters are devoted to the history of Soviet psychology in the textbooks written by Misiak and Sexton (1966), Murphy and Kovach (1972), and Sahakian (1975).

To Test or Not to Test?

In 1936, the psychometric approach to individual differences was declared, ex officio, unacceptable in the Soviet Union, being "founded on pseudoscientific experiments and on an endless number of senseless and harmful research questionnaires and tests...condemned by the Party." The trends in the Soviet views on these matters were characterized (Brožek, 1972a) by a shift from "tests" to collections of destandardized and de-quantified "tasks" (zadanie), an attempt to develop a 'Pavlovian' variety of psychometrics and, eventually, a call for a reexamination (peresmotr) of the issue in view of the pressing need for economic techniques that would provide information of a subject's mental niveau.

Physiology and Psychology

Physiology of behavior and psychology are considered at substantial length in Graham's discipline-by-discipline account (1974, 1st ed. 1966). Special attention is given to the physiologists Pavlov and Anokhin, and the psychologists Vygotskii and Rubinshtein. The important 1962 conference on The Philosophical Problems of the Physiology of Higher Nervous Activity and Psychology, held in Moscow, is considered in detail.

The proceedings are characterized as "the best single source
for an understanding of the philosophic issues in Soviet
physiology and psychology since the passing of the Stalinist
era" (p. 391).

T. R. Payne on S. L. Rubinshtein

Payne's book is the only monograph in the history of
Soviet psychology to appear in English in the 1960s (Payne,
1968; cf. Brozek, 1970a). Its first three sections are
closer to the "historical" pole, the last three sections,
to the "philosophical" pole.

Presentation of the life and literary activity of
Rubinshtein is preceded by a section on "The Sources of
Soviet Psychological Theory," in physiology (Sechenov,
Bekhterev, Pavlov) and in Marxist-Leninist philosophy, and
on "The Development of Psychological Theory in the Soviet
Union."

Payne divides the history of Soviet psychology into
three major periods labeled 'mechanist' (1917-1930),
'dialectical' (1930-1950), and 'Pavlovian' (since 1950).
This reflects the changes, over the years, in the requirements for a truly 'Marxist' psychology. During the early
nineteen-twenties, the chief requirement was that it be
materialist. In the nineteen-thirties dialectics was added,
followed in 1950 by the addition of Pavlovian physiology
(Payne, 1968, p. 62).

Payne's appraisal regarding the effects of extrinsic
ideological pressures is negative. The Party's insistence,
in the 1930s, that psychology be rebuilt on the basis of
Marxism-Leninism

> "has meant not only mere adherence to its prin-
> ciples but even to the very words used by the
> 'classics' (of Marxism-Leninism) when referring
> to psychological subjects. This has acted as a
> brake on the normal development of psychological
> theory, has forced Soviet psychology into a
> theoretical straightjacket and produced a vast
> crop of purely exegetical problems." (Payne,
> 1968, p. 168).

The added dogmatic insistence in the early 1950s that psychology be faithful not only to Marx and Lenin but to Pavlov as well, and to do so undeviatingly, compounded the confusion.

In keeping with the general periodization of Soviet psychology, Payne portrays Rubinshtein's share in the 're-construction' (perestroika) of the philosophical foundations of Soviet psychology, first on the basis of Marxist-Leninist dialectical unity of consciousness and behavior, and then (since 1950), by incorporating some general aspects of Pav-lov's physiology of higher nervous activity. These themes are developed in the two closing sections analyzing Rubin-shtein's views on the twofold relationship of the mind to the material world, the outer and the inner. The mind is viewed as the ideal reflection of the external reality as well as a function of the brain (highest nervous activity).

The presentation is thoroughly documented. The mono-graph is provided with a subject and name index, a selective bibliography of publications in Russian as well as in the major Western languages, principally English, and a list of books and articles by Rubinshtein.

East and West in Parallel and in Comparison

The "comparative encyclopedia" on Marxism, Communism and Western Society gives consideration also to the field of psychology. The account of the developments in the West and in the Soviet Union (Kussmann, 1973) is supplemented by direct comparisons of several aspects, including scientific societies and philosophical considerations (Brožek, 1973). The topic was presented in a more comprehensive manner else-where (Brožek, 1971).

Razraniana

Gregory Razran, for many years associated with the Department of Psychology of Queens College, has been an ex-perimentalist, a theoretician and, almost reluctantly and "on the margin", a historian. While Razran considered in several contexts the Soviet contributions with reference to developments in the USA (Razran, 1965), his opus magnum is the monograph Mind in Evolution (1971). The author acknow-ledges his debt to I. P. Pavlov's approach to the study and interpretation of learned behavior ("higher nervous activity") but is appreciative also of the major contributions made by Sechenov, Ukhtomskii, Beritashvili, and Anokhin. His aim, expressed in the book's subtitle, is "An East-West Synthesis of Learned Behavior and Cognition."

Pavloviana in the USA

Efforts are being made to locate, examine and register the archival materials related to the life of I. P. Pavlov and held outside the Soviet Union, particularly in the United States. The first installment refers to the holdings of the Archives of the History of American Psychology, University of Akron (Brožek and McPherson, 1973). While the Archives contain at present no letters exchanged between Pavlov and the American scientists, the correspondence among American psychologists (incl. Lashley, Yerkes, and J. B. Watson) contains informative references to Pavlov. Additional references to Pavlov have been located in a variety of other sources, including reminiscences of psychologists and R. M. Yerkes "obituary" of Pavlov, written in 1916. There are still photographs and motion picture films portraying Pavlov and some of his close associates.

Rahmani's Survey

In Rahmani's (1973) account of Soviet psychology, emphasizing the events and achievements of the last two decades, the introductory chapter (pp. 5-60) provides an overview of developments from 1917 to 1950. The Soviet views on the nature of the mind are discussed in extenso (pp. 61-124). Among the specific research topics, two are treated in depth: sensory cognition, and thought and language. Less extensive treatment is accorded to memory. Brief chapters are devoted to personality and the related topics of affective processes and motivation ("will").

Except for the historical introduction, the author's approach is "developmental" rather than "historical", in a traditional sense. The focus is on the theories of scientific psychology, considered in relation to experimental findings and the metatheoretical (philosophical, "methodological" -- in Soviet terminology) issues and positions.

Soviet Psychology on the Upswing

In his analysis of selected aspects of contemporary
Soviet psychology (conditioned reflexes, cognitive processes,
child development, and orienting reactions), Molino (1969)
stresses that, following the death of Stalin in 1953, important innovations in experimental research and shifts of
theoretical emphasis have taken place. He gives a "yes"
answer to the question "Is there a new Soviet psychology?"

An account of Soviet psycholinguistics was contributed
by Prŭcha (1972).

A section of recent developments in Soviet psychology
was incorporated into an overview of the world-wide scene
(Brožek and Rahmani, 1975). The following research areas
are considered: neurocybernetics, perception, thinking and
language, psychology of personality, and social psychology.
A quantitative portrait of current research interests is
based on the analysis of the content of the Fourth Congress
of the Soviet Psychology Society, held in Tbilisi, Georgia,
on 21-24 June 1971. The chapter closes with the presentation
of the Soviet psychologists' view of the challenges of tomorrow.

PART II. SOVIET AUTHORS

"Soviet Psychology", a Journal of Translations

The principal vehicle of information, in English, on
contemporary psychology in the USSR is the journal Soviet
Psychology, initially combined with psychiatry (Soviet Psychology and Psychiatry, Vol. 1, 1963). In 1967 it began a
separate existence. The journal's principal function is to
publish translations of selected current journal articles.
At times a whole issue is devoted to a specific topic, such
as psycholinguistics (Slobin, 1969), experimental neuroses
(Cole and Bowden, 1969/70), and Soviet research on primates
(Cole and Bowden, 1970). Additional special topics included perception and learning (Vol. 10, 1971), social psychology (Vol. 11, No. 1, 1972), and psychophysiology (Vol. 12,
No. 3, 1973; cf. Mecacci and Brožek, 1973).

Honoring Bekhterev and Vygotskii

V. M. Bekhterev (1857-1927) and L. S. Vygotskii (1896-1932) are among the greatest of Russian and Soviet psychologists.

It was appropriate that a special issue of Soviet Psychology, edited by M. Cole (1969), was devoted to V. M. Bekhterev's "developmental reflexology", one of the leading research areas in the 1920s, later largely erased from the Soviet scene on ideological grounds. Cole (1969a) contributed the introduction. The paper, by Bekhterev and Shchelovanov (1969), on the establishment of the objective (reflexological) study of child development was first published, in Russian, in 1925.

A reprint of Bekhterev's General Principles of Human Reflexology, with an introductory note by L. Rahmani, was made available recently (Bechterev, 1973). The translation was first published in 1932.

The Vygotskii Memorial Issue of Soviet Psychology (Slobin, 1967) contains a preface by Jerome S. Bruner; translations of Vygotskii's lecture on the role of play in the development of the child, given in 1933 and published a third of a century later (Vygotskii, 1967); papers on Vygotskii's significance for the study of perception (Zaporozhets, 1967), the concept of internalization of external activity as a crucial process in the genesis of mental activity (Gal'perin, 1967), the relation between teaching and mental development (El'konin, 1967), the problem of generalization (Davydov, 1967), and localization of brain functions (Luriya, 1967); and a bibliography of Vygotskii's publications (Slobin, 1967a).

Bruner (p. 5) views Vygotskii as "an important link between Soviet psychology and contemporary American psychology -- a link at the cognitive pole, just as Pavlov was at the stimulus-response conditioning pole."

Fifty Years of Psychology in the USSR

Three special issues of Soviet Psychology have been devoted to translations of papers reviewing the developments during the years 1917-1967 (Brožek, 1968, 1968/1969). The basic fields of psychology in the Soviet Union, the applied fields, and the Georgian studies on "set" were taken up, in turn. These materials, to which an expanded introduction and translations of additional articles have been added, were published in a book form (Brožek and Slobin, 1972). The basic fields include general psychology, physiology of higher nervous activity, psychophysiology, research on vision, neuropsychology, and developmental psychology. The applied fields encompass the psychology of education (upbringing and instruction), industrial psychology, aviation and space psychology, military psychology, and the psychology of sports.

The fact that in the past the development of psychology in the Soviet Union has been uneven was noted by Lomov (1972, p. 347): "While educational psychology has received wide attention in this country, medical and forensic (law) psychology are relatively neglected; much is being done in engineering psychology and significantly less in social psychology (although the importance of the latter is growing continually); the problems of animal psychology, etc., scarcely receive any attention at all."

S. L. Rubinshtein on Post-War Developments in Soviet Psychology

On the initiative of UNESCO, the USSR Academy of Sciences prepared a report, published in English, on the work done in the USSR in "social sciences" during the first 15 years or so following the Second World War. S. L. Rubinshtein, a Corresponding Member of the USSR Academy of Sciences, was asked to write the section on psychology (Rubinštejn, 1965). Materials pertaining to the year 1960 were contributed by E. A. Budilova. A brief consideration is given to general (theoretical) psychology. The second part of the chapter deals with research in the areas of sensation and perception, memory, speech and thought, personality, aptitudes, comparative psychology, human development, educational psychology, and the psychology of sports.

Out of the total of 42 volumes cited by Rubinshtein (1965), 13 were published during 1946-1950, 7 in 1951-1955, and 22 in the period 1956-1960. Some of the works cited came from the pen of scientists who regarded themselves as anthropologists (and had interest in the behavior of anthropoid apes) and physiologists.

A Soviet Anthology

In connection with the 1966 International Congress of Psychology, held in Moscow, an anthology was brought out by Leont'ev, Luriya, and Smirnov (1966). The aim of this collection of articles was to acquaint foreign readers with Soviet research in psychology and some related disciplines.

It consists of two parts, entitled "General Problems of Psychology and Psychophysiology", and "Sensations, Perception", respectively. While the second part is fairly homogeneous, the first part includes papers that would not be regarded as "psychology" in the Soviet Union. One, written by E. A. Asratyan, is entitled plainly "The Physiology of Conditioned Reflex".

Cole-Maltzman's "Handbook"

The Handbook (1969; cf. Brožek, 1970) consists of four parts devoted, respectively, to developmental psychology, abnormal and social psychology, general experimental psychology and research on the physiological bases of behavior. Underrepresented is the work on sensation and perception, and the vast literature on the learning of specific school subjects. The psychology of sports, which is one of the specialties of Soviet psychology, and research on space flight are missin

The editors provided an informative section on "Historical Background" in their general Introduction, wrote introductions to all the individual papers, and provided footnotes These features help importantly to place in perspective the information provided by the Soviet authors. The editors succeeded in their hope that "historical and theoretical background information of this kind...should make the individual studies more understandable than they would otherwise be if read in isolation" (op. cit., p. XI). This is a good example of the "service role" of historiography to contemporary research, a role that may be disdained by those stressing "history for history's sake" but that, in this reviewer's opinion, represents a valuable contribution of history.

Soviet Contributions to an American Book on the History of Psychology

Soviet authors contributed three essays to the volume on Historical Roots of Contemporary Psychology, edited by

Wolman (1968). They deal, respectively, with I. M. Sechenov
(Yaroshevskii, 1968), I. P. Pavlov (Anokhin, 1968), and L.
S. Vygotskii (Leont'ev and Luria, 1968). The omission of
V. M. Bekhterev (1857-1927) is unfortunate.

Soviet Books in Translation

The account of the "contemporary" scene in Soviet
psychology (Brožek, 1973), appended to the Marx-Hillix
Systems and Theories of Psychology, is focused on some 25
Soviet monographs translated into English and published
commercially outside the Soviet Union.

Additional translations deal with aphasia (Luria, 1970),
electrophysiology of the nervous system (Rusinov, 1970), memory (Beritashvili, 1971), neuroanatomy of the visual system
(Shkol'nik-Yarros, 1971), effects of brain lesions (Luria,
1972), individual differences (Nebylitsyn, 1972; cf. also
Nebylitsyn and Gray, 1972), inner speech and thought (A. N.
Sokolov, 1972), visual images (Zinchenko and Vergiles, 1972),
clinical psychology (Zeigarnik, 1972; cf. Brožek and Rahmani,
1974), neuropsychology (Luria, 1974), and neurophysiology of
the conditioned reflex (Anokhin, 1974).

Sechenoviana

In Sechenov's Selected Works, first published in 1935,
the following items appeared in English translation: Reflexes of the Brain, Who Must Investigate the Problems of
Psychology and How, Impressions and Reality, and The Elements
of Thought. The section on Reflexes of the Brain was reprinted in the USA (Sechenov, 1965). The other three essays
together with the author's 1935 biography from the pen of
M. N. Shaternikov, are included in a recent American reprint
(Sechenov, 1973).

The 1965 edition of the essay Reflexes of the Brain,
first published in 1863, contains a biography of Sechenov by
Kh. S. Koshtoyants (pp. 119-139) and a postscript by W. A.
Rosenblith (pp. 143-145). Rosenblith underscores Sechenov's
concern with the nervous system as a control mechanism, antici-
pating Norbert Wiener's Cybernetics as the study of "control
and communication in the animal and the machine." In Rosenblith's formulation, Sechenov's "reflexological approach to
the understanding of behavior was a pioneering effort not

only in Russia but throughout the Western world" (p. 114).

Luria's Autobiography

The sixth volume of A History of Psychology in Autobiography, edited by Gardner Lindzey (1974), contains a retrospective analysis of the road traveled by A. R. Luria,
born in 1902 (1974a). The contribution is important on at
least two counts: First, the author's long and highly
productive professional career. Secondly, the focus on the
"description of the period in which the author lived and a
biography of the people who were decisive influences in the
development of psychological science of which he was a part"
(p. 254).

Relevant also are parts of the autobiography of the
Polish scientist, Jerzy Konorski, contained in the same
volume, referring to his work with Pavlov in Leningrad
(1931-1933) and his war-time years at the Primate Research
Center in Sukhumi, in the Caucasus (1940-1945).

The response of the Soviet scientists to Konorski's
1948 monograph Conditioned Reflexes and Neuron Organization
reflected the temper of the times. The pejorative label of
a "revisionist", applied to Konorski during the early Stalinist 1950s, was erased in the mid-1950s, following Stalin's
death.

BIBLIOGRAPHY

Introduction

BROŽEK, J. USSR: Current activities in the history of
physiology and psychology. Journal of the History
of Biology, 1971, 4, 185-208.

BROŽEK, J. Soviet psychology. I. In: H. J. Eysenck,
W. Arnold & R. Meili (Eds.), Encyclopedia of
Psychology. New York: Herder & Herder, 1972,
Vol. III, 248-251.

BROŽEK, J. Soviet historiography of psychology. I. Sources
of biographic and bibliographic information. Journal
of the History of the Behavioral Sciences, 1973, 9,
152-161; II. Contributions of non-Russian authors,
ibid., 1973a, 9, 213-216; III. Between philosophy and
history, ibid., 1974, 10, 195-201; IV. History of
psychology abroad, ibid., 1974a, 10, 348-351.

LURIA, A. R. Soviet psychology. II. In: H. J. Eysenck,
W. Arnold, & R. Meili (Eds.), Encyclopedia of
Psychology. New York: Herder & Herder, 1972,
Vol. III, 251-253.

MECACCI, L. Soviet Psychology in the Western Countries.
Rome, Italy: Institute of Psychology, National
Research Council, 1971.

Part I.

ANONYMOUS. Noted figures in the history of Soviet
psychology: Pictures and brief biographies. Soviet
Psychology and Psychiatry, 1966, 4, (3-4), 105-112.

BOWDEN, D. & COLE, M. Glossary of terms frequently
encountered in Soviet psychology. Soviet Psychology
and Psychiatry, 1966, 4, (3-4), 10-15.

BROŽEK, J. Contemporary Soviet psychology. Transactions
of the New York Academy of Sciences, 1965, Series 2,
27, 422-438.

BROŽEK, J. Contemporary Soviet psychology. In: N.
    O'Connor, (Ed.), Present-day Russian Psychology.
    New Hork: Pergamon Press, 1966, 178-198.

BROŽEK, J. Organizational structure of the Soviet
    Psychological Society. American Psychologist, 1967,
    22, 451.

BROŽEK, J. Toward a history of Soviet psychology: A set
    of bibliographies. Soviet Psychology, 1968, 6 (3-4),
    8-12.

BROŽEK, J. Review of A. V. Petrovskii, "Istoriya sovetskoi
    psikhologii" (History of Soviet psychology) and
    M. G. Yaroshevskii, "Istoriya psikhologii" (History of
    psychology). Contemporary Psychology, 1969, 14,
    432-434.

BROŽEK, J. Essay review of Razvitie biologii v SSSR
    (Development of biology in the USSR). Journal of the
    History of Biology, 1969a, 2, 439-444.

BROŽEK, J. Soviet psychology's coming of age. American
    Psychologist, 1970, 25, 1057-1058.

BROŽEK, J. Review of T. R. Payne, "S. L. Rubinštejn and the
    philosophical foundations of Soviet psychology."
    Russian Review, 1970, 29, 350-351.

BROŽEK, J. USSR: Current activities in the history of
    physiology and psychology. Journal of the History
    of Biology, 1971, 4, 185-208.

BROŽEK, J. Recent Russian Pavloviana. Conditional
    Reflex. 1971a, 6 157-165.

BROŽEK, J. Soviet and American psychology: Comparison
    and comments (in English). In: T. Kussmann and
    J. Brožek, "Die Lehr- und Forschungsgebiete der
    Psychologie im internationalen Vergleich."
    Berichte des Bundesinstituts für ostwissenschaftliche
    und internationale Studien (Köln), 1971b, 61-93,
    129-134.

BROŽEK, J. Soviet writings of the 1960's on the history of
    psychology and the physiology of behavior. History of
    Science, 1972, 10, 56-87.

BROŽEK, J. To test or not to test: Trends in the Soviet
    views. Journal of the History of the Behavioral
    Sciences, 1972a, 8, 243-248.

BROŽEK, J. Psychology: C. Comparative remarks on Soviet
    and U. S. Psychology. In: C. D. Kernig (Ed.),
    Marxism, Communism and Western Society: A Comparative
    Encyclopedia. New York: Herder & Herder, Vol. 7,
    1973, 105-110, 112-113.

BROŽEK, J. Essay Review: Six recent additions to the
    history of physiology in the USSR. Journal of the
    History of Biology, 1973a, 6, 317-334.

BROŽEK, J. West-German sovietica. Contemporary Psychology,
    1975, 20, 310-311.

BROŽEK, J. & HERZ, A. PIRSCENOK. Recent Russian books in
    psychology. Contemporary Psychology, 1974, 19,
    421-426.

BROŽEK, J. & HOSKOVEC, J. Current Soviet psychology: A
    systematic review. Soviet Psychology and Psychiatry,
    1966, 4, (3-4), 16-44.

BROŽEK, J. & HOSKOVEC, J. Soviet psychology in English:
    Translations of books. Soviet Psychology and
    Psychiatry, 1966a, 4, (3-4), 100-104.

BROŽEK, J. & HOSKOVEC, J. Sovietica in English: In the
    press, in the works, on the drawing board.
    Contemporary Psychology, 1966b, 11, 382-383.

BROŽEK, J., HOSKOVEC, J., & SLOBIN, D. I. Reviews in
    English of recent Soviet psychology: A bibliography.
    Soviet Psychology and Psychiatry, 1966, 4, (3-4),
    95-99.

BROŽEK, J. & MECACCI, L. New Soviet research institute.
    American Psychologist, 1974, 29, 475-478.

BROŽEK, J. & McPHERSON, MARION WHITE. Pavloviana in the
    USA: Archives of the History of American Psychology,
    University of Akron. Conditional Reflex, 1973, 8,
    236-244.

BROŽEK, J. & RAHMANI, L. Soviet psychology on the upswing.
    In H. Misiak & V. Stand & Sexton (Eds.), Psychology
    Around the World. Monterey, Cal.: Brooks/Cole, 1975
    (in press).

GRAHAM, R. L. Physiology and psychology. In: Science and
    Philosophy in the Soviet Union. New York: Vintage
    Books (Random House), 1974 (1st ed., 1966), 355-429.

GRAY, J. A. Attention, consciousness and voluntary control
    of behavior in Soviet psychology: Philosophical roots
    and research branches. In: N. O'Connor (Ed.), Present-
    Day Russian Psychology, 1966, 1-38.

KIRMAN, B. H. Psychotherapy in the Soviet Union. In: N.
    O'Connor (Ed.), Present-Day Russian Psychology, 1966,
    39-62.

KUSSMAN, T. Psychology. A. Western. B. Soviet.
    In: C. D. Kernig (Ed.), Marxism, Communism and
    Western Society: A Comparative Encyclopedia. New
    York: Herder & Herder, Vol. 7, 1973, 90-104, 110-112.

LYNN, R. Abnormal psychology in the USSR. In: N. O'Connor
    (Ed.), Present-Day Russian Psychology, 1966, 92-108.

LYNN, R. Attention, Arousal and Orientation Reaction.
    Oxford, England: Pergamon Press, 1966a.

MISIAK, H. & SEXTON, VIRGINIA S. History of Psychology:
    An Overview. New York: Grune & Stratton, 1966,
    258-280.

MURPHY, G. AND KOVACH, J. K. Historical Introduction to
    Modern Psychology. 3rd ed. New York: Harcourt,
    Brace & Jovanovich, 1972, 377-398.

MOLINO, J. A. Is there a new Soviet psychology? In: A.
    Smirenko (Ed.), Social Thought in the Soviet Union.
    Chicago Quadrangle Books, 1969, 300-327.

O'CONNOR, N. Present-Day Russian Psychology: A Symposium by Seven Authors. Oxford, England: Pergamon Press, 1966.

PAYNE, T. R. S. L. Rubinstejn and the Philosophical Foundations of Soviet Psychology. Dordrecht (Holland): Reidel & New York: Humanities Press, 1968.

PRŮCHA, J. Soviet Psycholinguistics. The Hague: Mouton, 1972.

RABBITT, P. M. A. Some statistical and cybernetic models in recent Soviet psychology. In: N. O'Connor (Ed.), Present-Day Russian Psychology, 1966, 63-91.

RAHMANI, L. Review of F. N. Fedoseev (Chief Ed.), "Filosofskie voprosy," Contemporary Psychology, 1965, 10, 249-250.

RAHMANI, L. Studies on the mental development of the child. In: N. O'Connor (Ed.), Present-Day Russian Psychology, 1966, 152-178.

RAHMANI, L. Soviet Psychology: Philosophical, Theoretical and Experimental Issues. New York: International Universities Press, 1973.

RAZRAN, G. Russian physiologists' psychology and American experimental psychology: A historical and a systematic collation and a look into the future. Psychological Bulletin, 1965, 53, 42-64.

RAZRAN, G. Mind in Evolution: An East-West Synthesis of Learned Behavior and Cognition. Boston: Houghton Mifflin, 1971.

SAHAKIAN, W. S. History and Systems of Psychology. New York: Wiley, 1975, 377-409.

SCHULTZ, D. A History of Modern Psychology. New York: Academic Press, 1975, 2nd ed.

SLOBIN, D. I. (Ed.), Handbook of Soviet psychology, oviet Psychology and Psychiatry, 1966, 4, (3-4), 1-146.

SLOBIN, D. I.   Directory of Soviet institutions engaged in
    psychological, psychophysiological, and psychiatric
    research.   Soviet Psychology and Psychiatry, 1966,
    4, (3-4), 113-119.

SLOBIN, D. I.   Soviet psycholinguistics.   In: N. O'Connor
    (Ed.), Present-Day Russian Psychology, 1966,
    109-151.

SLOBIN, D. A.   Articles on history of psychology appearing
    in "Voprosy psikhologii" since its inception in
    1955.   Soviet Psychology, 1968, 6, (304), 13-18.

SLOBIN, D. I. & GORDON, B. A.   Directory of Soviet
    scientists engaged in psychological and psychophysio-
    logical research.   Soviet Psychology and Psychiatry,
    1966, 4, (3-4), 120-144.

WATSON, R. I.   The Great Psychologists from Aristotle to
    Freud.   2nd ed.   Philadelphia: Lippincott, 1968.

Part II

ANOKHIN, P. K.   Ivan P. Pavlov and psychology.   In: B. B.
    Wolman (Ed.), Historical Roots of Contemporary
    Psychology, 1968, 131-159.

ANOKHIN, P. K.   Biology and Neurophysiology of the
    Conditioned Reflex and its Role in Adaptive Behavior.
    Trans. from Russian by S. A. Corson.   New York:
    Pergamon Press, 1974.

BECHTEREV, V. M.   General Principles of Human Reflexology.
    New York: Arno Press, 1973.   (Reprint of the 1932
    edition published by International Publishers,
    New York).

BEKHTEREV, V. M. & SHCHELOVANOV, N. M.   Toward the
    establishment of a developmental reflexology.   Soviet
    Psychology, 1969, 8 (1), 7-25.

BERITASHVILI, I. S.   Vertebrate Memory: Characteristics
    and Origin.   New York: Plenum Press, 1971.

BROŽEK, J. Review of B. Simon and Joan Simon (Eds.), Educational psychology in the USSR, Slavic and East European Journal, 1965, 9, 227-228.

BROŽEK, J. Russian contributions on brain and behavior. Science, 1966, 152, 930-932.

BROŽEK, J. (Ed.), Fifty years of Soviet psychology: An historical perspective. Soviet Psychology, 1968, 6, (3-4), 1-128; 1968, 7, (1), 1-72.

BROŽEK, J. (Ed.), Special issue on Georgian psychology. Soviet Psychology, 1968/69, 7, (2), 1-55.

BROŽEK, J. Review of M. Cole and I. Maltzman (Eds.), A Handbook of Contemporary Soviet Psychology. Contemporary Psychology, 1970, 15, 436-438.

BROŽEK, J. Soviet psychology. Appendix B to M. H. Marx and W. A. Hillix, Systems and Theories in Psychology, 2nd ed. New York, McGraw-Hill, 1973, 521-548.

BROŽEK, J. & RAHMANI, L. Pathopsychology. Contemporary Psychology, 1974, 19, 215-216.

BROŽEK, J. & SLOBIN, D. Psychology in the USSR: An Historical Perspective. White Plains, New York: International Arts and Sciences Press, 1972.

COLE, M. (Ed.), Special issue on V. M. Bekhterev's developmental reflexology. Soviet Psychology, 1969, 8, (1), 1-78.

COLE, M. Introduction (to a special issue on V. M. Bekhterev's developmental reflexology). Soviet Psychology, 1969a, 8, (1), 3-6.

COLE, M. & BOWDEN, D. (Eds.), Experimental neuroses. Soviet Psychology, 8, (2), 83-168, 1969/70.

COLE, M. & BOWDEN, D. (Eds.), Soviet research on primates. Soviet Psychology, 9, (1), 1-102, 1970.

COLE, M. & MALTZMAN, I. (Eds.), A Handbook of Contemporary
    Soviet Psychology. Translated from the Russian by
    Rosa Glickman, D. G. Nichols, Elka Schuman & Lynn
    Solotaroff. New York: Basic Books, 1969.

DAVYDOV, V. V. The problem of generalization in the works
    of L. S. Vygotsky. Soviet Psychology, 1967, 5,
    (3), 42-52.

EL'KONIN, D. B. The problem of instruction and development
    in the works of L. S. Vygotsky. Soviet Psychology,
    1967, 5, (3), 34-41.

GAL'PERIN, P. YA. On L. S. Vygotsky's notion of
    internalization. Soviet Psychology, 1967, 5, (3),
    28-33.

KONORSKI, J. Jerzy Konorski. In: G. Lindzey (Ed.),
    A History of Psychology in Autobiography, Vol. VI.
    Englewood Cliffs, New Jersey: Prentice-Hall 1974,
    185-217.

LEONT'EV, A. N. & LURIYA, A. R. The psychological ideas
    of L. S Vygotskii. In: B. B. Wolman (Ed.),
    Historical Roots of Contemporary Psychology, 1968,
    336-337.

LEONT'EV, A., LURIYA, A., & SMIRNOV, A. (Eds.),
    Psychological Research in the USSR (in English).
    Moscow: Progress Publishers, 1966.

LOMOV, B. F. Present status and future developments of
    psychology in the USSR in the light of the decisions
    of the 24th congress of the CPSU. Soviet Psychology,
    1972, 10, 329-358.

LURIA (LURIYA), A. R. L. S. Vygotsky and the problem of
    functional localization. Soviet Psychology, 1967,
    5, (3), 53-57.

LURIA, A. R. Traumatic Aphasia: Its Syndromes,
    Psychology and Treatment. The Hague: Mouton, 1970.

LURIA, A. R. The Man with a Shattered World: A History
    of a Brain Wound. New York: Basic Books, 1972.

LURIA, A. R. The Working Brain: An Introduction to
    Neuropsychology. Trans. from Russian by B. Haigh.
    New York: Basic Books, 1974.

LURIA, A. R. A. R. Luria. In: G. Lindzey (Ed.), A
    History of Psychology in Autobiography, Vol. VI.
    Englewood Cliffs, New Jersey: Prentice-Hall, 1974a,
    251-292.

MECACCI, L. & BROŽEK, J. Soviet psychophysiology:
    Introduction. Soviet Psychology, 1973, 11, (3),
    4-22.

NEBYLITSYN, V. D. Fundamental Properties of the Human
    Nervous System. New York: Plenum Press, 1972.

NEBYLITSYN, V. D., & GRAY, J. A. (Eds.). Biological Basis
    of Human Behavior. New York: Academic Press, 1972.

RUSINOV, V. S. (Ed.) Electrophysiology of the Central
    Nervous System. New York: Plenum Press, 1970.

SECHENOV, I. M. Reflexes of the Brain. Translated from
    Russian by S. Belsky; first published in 1863.
    Cambridge, Mass.: MIT Press, 1965.

SECHENOV, I. M. Biographical Sketch and Essays. New York:
    Arno Press, 1973.

SHKOL'NIK-YARROS, EKATERINA G. Neurons and Interneuronal
    Connections of the Central Visual System. New York:
    Plenum Press, 1971.

SLOBIN, D. A. (Ed.), Vygotsky Memorial issue. Soviet
    Psychology, 5, (3), 1-60, 1967.

SLOBIN, D. I. Bibliography of L. S. Vygotsky. Soviet
    Psychology, 1967a, 5, (3), 58-60.

SLOBIN, D. I. Articles on history of psychology appearing
    in Voprosy psikhologii since its inception in 1955.
    Soviet Psychology, 1968, 6, (3-4), 13-18.

SLOBIN, D. I. (Ed.), Special issue on Soviet psycho-
    linguistics. Soviet Psychology, 7, (3), 1-56, 1969.

SOKOLOV, A. N. Inner Speech and Thought. New York:
    Plenum Press, 1972.

VYGOTSKY, L. S. Play and its role in the mental
    development of the child. Soviet Psychology, 1967,
    5, (3), 6-18. The original written in 1933.

WOLMAN, B. B. (Ed.), Historical Roots of Contemporary
    Psychology. New York: Harper and Row, 1968.

YAROSHEVSKII, M. G. I. M. Sechenov--The founder of
    objective psychology. In: B. B. Wolman (Ed.),
    Historical Roots of Contemporary Psychology,
    1968, 77-110.

ZAPOROZHETS, A. V. L. S. Vygotsky's role in the study of
    the problems of perception. Soviet Psychology, 1967,
    5, (3), 19-27.

ZEIGARNIK, B. V. Experimental Abnormal Psychology.
    New York: Plenum Press, 1972.

ZINCHENKO, V. P., & VERGILES, N. YU. Formation of
    Visual Images: Studies on Stabilized Retinal Images.
    New York: Consultants Bureau, 1972.

SOCIAL PSYCHOLOGY IN THE SOVIET UNION:

SOME COMMENTS

Robert M. Krauss

Department of Psychology

Columbia University

One of my favorite writers, the late A. J. Liebling, political analyst, social critic, sports reporter, gastronome, and general know-it-all, once wrote something that seems particularly relevant to my presence here today. He was speaking of newspaper reporters and what he said is:

> There are three kinds of writers of news in our generation. In inverse order of wordly consideration they are: (1) the reporter who writes what he sees; (2) the interpretive reporter who writes what he sees and what he construes to be its meaning; and (3) the expert, who writes what he construes to be the meaning of what he hasn't seen (Liebling, 1961, p. 225).

As regards social psychology in the Soviet Union (and unlike my fellow panelists, I am an expert only in Liebling's sense), I am prepared to discuss the significance of that which I haven't seen. My knowledge of this topic is based almost totally on what I have read and I have not read a great deal. Indeed, the only justification I can give for being here at all is that I know more about it than do most of my fellow social psychologists. And that fact, I think, contains a lesson of some interest.

While most researchers in child development, classical conditioning or psychophysiology know at least something about work in their area being done in the Soviet Union, I think it is fair to say that relatively few American social

psychologists can so much as name one of their Russian counterparts. In part, this is due to the fact that up until
rather recently the American version of social psychology,
and a single aspect of it at that, has been the dominant
focus for social psychologists the Western world over. This
is not to say that there were not, in the 1950s and early
1960s, other social psychologies. Certainly there were--in
the USA as well as abroad--and very likely their adherents
collectively outnumbered those in the American experimental-
ist tradition. But none of these orientations individually
had anywhere near the prominence that the American approach
did--again either here or abroad. At least in decades past,
American experimental social psychologists tended to feel
that there was little point in studying the social psychology of Nation X when a good portion of Nation X's social
psychologists were in this country learning to work in our
tradition. And if that attitude was both arrogant and
myopic, which it was, it was not totally without a foundation in reality. Most Americans knew the work of their
Western European counterparts well, often as a result of
having served as their collaborators and mentors.

Not so for the Soviet Union. For a variety of reasons,
American social psychologists have had few contacts in the
USSR and know little of the work being done there. It is
tempting to blame this on the Cold War, but that would, I
think, be an oversimplification. The Cold War may have made
it difficult for Russian and American researchers in, say,
conditioning to share their knowledge, but it did not totally prevent those who were genuinely motivated from doing
so. I think the source lies in two circumstances.

First, if political ideology can affect psychology as
it can all of science, it seems to me the study of man's
social nature would be particularly susceptible. Certainly
in the Soviet Union, where a technical question in genetics
was capable of developing into a political cause célebre,
theories of social behavior tainted by alien political
ideology could be a dangerous bit of baggage. Let me
hasten to add that the situation is perfectly symmetrical.
I cannot recall any social psychologists in the USA in
the 1950s doing experimental work or much of any work
that derived from a Marxist orientation, however remotely.
So far as I know, no one was called before Senator McCarthy

committee for studying Pavlovian conditioning on a federal
grant, but I'm not sure that this sort of immunity would have
extended to a study entitled, "A Marxist Leninist Approach
to Conflict Resolution." So the barriers to effective
communication were both formidable and bidirectional.

There is also a second, and considerably less complicated factor. To put it simply, there really wasn't much
that an American social psychologist would recognize as
social psychology in the USSR prior to the 1950s.

There is something of an irony here. Given the Russian
ideological emphasis on the importance of social determinants of human affairs and their tendency to minimize the
importance of genetic explanations, one would expect social
psychology to occupy a central role in their investigations
of human behavior. And in a sense it does. Much Soviet
psychology, although not explicitly social psychology,
strongly emphasizes social determinants of behavior. Good
examples of this can be seen in the work of Vygotskii,
Leont'ev and Luria, familiar to most of us. But the study
of what specifically we have in mind as social psychology--
the empirical study of attitude change, social determinants
of personality and values, group problem solving and the
like--is less than two decades old.

It may come as something of a surprise then to note
that another and quite different social psychology existed
in post-Revolutionary Russia, using the conditioned reflex
as the primary explanatory concept. So eminent an investigator as Bekhterev in 1921 published a book entitled
Collective Reflexology (Bekhterev, 1921) that attempted to
reduce the laws of mass psychology to fundamental physical
laws, such as Newton's laws of motion. Viewing man as
preeminently a physiological creature, Bekhterev similarly
viewed society as a rather simple physiological mechanism.
The approach was no more successful that similar ill-
conceived attempts in the West to explain social behavior on
the basis of such monlithic concepts as instinct, habit,
or imitation. Probably the reflexological approach was
pushed to its furthest and most fanciful extreme by
Vasil'ev, who attempted to explain the American Civil War in
terms of the concept of inhibition. I cannot resist reading
to you a brief excerpt from his argument.

> The Civil War in the USA occurred because
> an inhibitory response to slavery developed
> in inhabitants of the Northern states. In
> this inhibited condition, they set about
> fighting the uninhibited inhabitants of
> the Southern states. But in the end,
> the great slaughter caused inhibitions
> even in the latter. When both were
> sufficiently inhibited, slavery dis-
> appeared and events thereafter ensued
> peacefully (Vasil'ev, 1927).

The reflexological approach was not the only social psychology developed in the post-Revolutionary period, but apparently none of these others fared much better. And so for about three decades social psychology in the Soviet Union remained an underdeveloped area. The interesting question is "Why?"

Explorations in the history of science are never straightforward and, for someone as unsophisticated in these matters as I am, they are a perilous enterprise indeed. The best I can do is to cite the explanation offered by A. V. Petrovskiy (1972) in his essay "The Emergence and Development of Social Psychology as a Science." Petrovskiy's explanation has a plausible ring to it and, in any event, it is interesting on other grounds.

The first reason, according to Petrovskiy, is the fact alluded to previously that post-Revolutionary general psychology was itself thought of as a social science, and hence the argument went that there was hardly a need for a special social psychology. And certainly the situation was not helped by the domination of what social psychology there was by the reflexologists, whose dismissal of any distinction between the human person and the biological organism, and indeed between man and society, was simply unacceptable.

A second reason that Petrovskiy offers is the recurring fear that "...social psychology would lead to a tendency in the study of historical events to replace historical materialism by a psychologizing of historical phenomena" (p. 17). I am not sufficiently knowledgeable to judge the adequacy of Petrovskiy's explanation and I would very much like to hear someone who can speak to that point.

But true or not, there is one aspect of Petrovskiy's explanation that strikes me as intrinsically interesting, and that is the way in which scientific considerations and ideological considerations are merged. At least up until very recently, American social scientists have tended to think of their science as somehow value or ideology free. I think many of us now believe this to have been a naive viewpoint, but certainly the relation of political ideology to the practice of science is rather more implicit and subtle in this country, as compared to the USSR. Consider, for example, the following statement by Sherkovin taken from a scholarly article entitled, "Mass Media and their Role in Social Life." "The most important function of mass media in bourgeois societies is to subject the minds and feeling of people to a constant apologia for capitalism, its institutions, ideas, principles, traditions, unique lifestyle, etc., whereas under Socialism the objectives of communication are the cleansing of bourgeois idealist contamination from the mind of the proletariat" (Sherkovin, 1972, p. 78). Now I have no difficulty imagining an American social psychologist believing the converse of this proposition and I can even imagine it being expressed in his writing, but never in such explicit fashion. I will have occasion to return to this point later.

Social psychological research in the USSR can be partitioned into four broad categories:

(1) <u>Social psychological phenomena in large groups or in society</u>. Such phenomena would include the effects of the mass media, what we in this country would call attitude change and persuasion; the diffusion of rumor, fashion, and prejudice, etc. The social psychology of social class would be included here but Petrovskiy notes without further explanation that there has been essential lack of psychological research in this area.

(2) <u>The phenomena of small groups</u>. This category includes most of the phenomena that we here include under the rubric of group dynamics—leadership, cohesiveness, interpersonal relations, group status, group atmosphere, etc.

(3) Phenomena of special or specific groups.
Group behavior is the dominant focus of Soviet
social psychology and a distinction is drawn
between general processes of groups and the
properties of groups in specific situations or
circumstances. Such groups include the family,
school classes, work groups, military brigades,
and the like. It is my impression that this
is very much an applied social psychology and
overlaps considerably with what in this country
would be classified as industrial, organizational, and educational psychology.

(4) Social psychological factors in personality development. The Russians have been
particularly interested in the way socialization shapes values and attitudes. Given the
strong interest in group life noted above, it
is not surprising that the role of group experience in personality development is an
important area of investigation. To quote
Petrovskiy again, "The individual personality
becomes an object of social psychology when
it is viewed as part of a system of relations
with a group, and when those of its traits
and characteristics that are a projection of
these interrelations are studied" (Petrovskiy,
1972, p. 22).

It would be inappropriate for me to comment on specific
studies, but it may be helpful for gaining a more concrete
feeling for the work being done to contrast it in a rather
general and necessarily subjective fashion to social
psychology in this country.

First, Russian social psychology has a strong theoretical orientation and social psychological theory in the USSR
tends to be both broad and general, comparable in scope and
goal to that of such American theorists as Lewin, Hull, and
Tolman. It is characteristic that Sherkovin, in the article
on mass media I referred to previously, remarked, "It is no
accident that such a phenomenon has become the object of
theoretical thought." I am struck, because an American
social psychologist would certainly have written "...becomes
the object of research," and I think that difference is
not simply a difference in literary style. Beginning in the

late 1950s, social psychologists in the USA have increasingly turned away from such broadly-based general theories
to models of more modest scope, to what the sociologist
Robert Merton has termed "theories of the middle range"
(Merton, 1957). It will be interesting to see whether a
similar development occurs in the USSR in ensuing decades.

As was noted previously, interaction is a major focus
of Russian social psychological inquiry. Although this was
also true of work done in this country two decades ago,
more recently the emphasis here has shifted to investigation of individual psychological processes that have
consequences for social behavior--which also results in a
rather asocial social psychology. Incidentally, some
observers discern in the work of Western European social
psychology a shifting back to this earlier orientation
(Israel and Tajfel, 1972). In any case it will be interesting to observe the path of development that Soviet social
psychology takes. It is my impression that the clearest
contrast between American and Russian social psychology
lies in the area of methodology. The contrived laboratory
experiment of the sort that has in the past characterized
much, if not most, of American research is seldom employed
in the Soviet Union. Most of their studies seem to be
conducted in natural settings, either as field or natural
experiments or straight descriptive studies, gathering data
from observation and questionnaires as well as measuring
performance. Typically the designs of their studies are
simple. Elaborate statistical procedures are rarely used.

I think it is also fair to say that a great deal of what
is called social psychology in the USSR would be called
applied psychology in this country. Indeed, I have the
feeling that my Soviet counterparts would not accept this
distinction as very meaningful. It is not unusual for a
Russian social psychologist to assert quite explicitly in
his writings that the purpose of psychological investigation
is to further the goals of Soviet society. I simply do not
know enough about contemporary Russian society to judge the
extent to which such statements are simple rhetoric--an
automatic gesture one is compelled to make--or actually reflect deeply-felt convictions. I suspect there is some of
both. Either way, for the American social psychologist who
comes freshly upon it as I did, it has rather an off-putting
effect. One is, I think, apt to come away with a sense that

there is something vaguely indecent about so intimate a relation between ideology and science. Such a feeling is likely to result, at least in part, from the notion that Western social science has in some sense managed to remain ideology-free.

I think that such a position is untenable. It would no be hard to demonstrate that Western social science has traditionally been framed in terms of prevailing political ideology, has gained material support because of its compatibility with such doctrine and has served to reinforce and extend interests generated by ideological concern. Certainly there have been differences in the ways in which social science and political doctrine have been related in the USSR and the USA. But it would be unrealistic to deny that in both nations the relationship exists and that its effect on the way science is done is important. Perhaps, then, a lesson we can learn from our Russian colleagues, in addition to the substance of their investigations, is a clearer appreciation of the forces that shape their, and our own, science.

BIBLIOGRAPHY

BEKHTEREV, V. M. (1921). _Kollektivnaya refleksologiya_ (Collective Reflexology). Kolos.

ISRAEL, J. and H. TAJFEL, eds. (1972). _The Context of Social Psychology_. Academic Press.

MERTON, R. K. (1957). _Social Theory and Social Structure_. Free Press.

PETROVSKIY, A. V. (1972). Paths of development of social psychology in USSR. Soviet Psychology 11:8-28.

SHERKOVIN, Y. A. (1972). The mass media and their role in social life. Soviet Psychology 11:65-84.

VASIL'EV, S. (1927) _Kharakteristika mekhanicheskogo materializma "Dialektika prirody."_ 2nd edition. Vologo

THE LURIA BATTERY OF TESTS:

TECHNIQUES AND PHILOSOPHY

Elkhonon A. Goldberg

R. F. Kennedy Center for Research in Mental
Retardation and Human Development, Albert
Einstein College of Medicine, Bronx, New York

Neuropsychology in the USSR is one of the branches of psychology which has for a long time attracted the attention and curiosity of Western psychologists. To a large degree it is due to the stature of A. R. Luria, who has been an acknowledged leader in this area of research in the USSR for several decades. The trend-setting institutions for neuropsychologic research in the USSR are A. R. Luria's laboratories at the Department of Psychology, Moscow State University, and the Burdenko Institute of Neurosurgery, Moscow.

Areas of interest represented in these laboratories are extremely diverse. Roughly speaking, they concentrate around the following areas:

1. The refinement of neuropsychological (behavioral) methods of local brain lesion diagnostics.

2. The rehabilitation of imparied functions, mainly speech-related ones.

3. The delineation of electrophysiological correlates of various types of focal brain dysfunctions.

4. The elaboration, based on pathological data, of an understanding of the brain functional systems relationship to various types of normal behaviors.

This last area is essentially interrelated with item (1). Recent interests in this area concentrate mainly on the role of prefrontal parts of the brain in planning and control over behavior; the relationship of diencephalic structures to memory; and interhemispheric relations and the subdivision of functions between them.

5. The emergence of a relatively new interest in child neuropsychology, mainly in the context of the development of hemispheric functional lateralization.

6. The emergence of a relatively new interest in applying neuropsychological data and methods to the understanding of the normal microstructure of information processing (not to be confused with gross brain-behavior relations, localization of functions, which is quite a traditional area of neuropsychology).

The particular studies carried out deal both with the semantic aspects of normal information processing (the "languages" of representation) and "technological" aspects (the composite structure of information processors). Thus, models of speech comprehension and production have been developed based on aphasiology data; research of the "languages" of the memory encoding of visual information and verbal context has been carried out, based on various types of memory discrepancies which follow local brain lesions. An attempt to reconstruct and to model the operational structure of various types of control systems involved in normal information processing, based on experiments with prefrontal patients, may serve as another example of this approach.

When one is confronted with the goal of describing a scientific setting with a broad range of interests as described above, there is always a dilemma, whether to attempt to make a sketch of everything, which inevitably would be extremely superficial, or to concentrate on some particular issues which may reveal the philosophy underlying the whole range of research. Following the second line, a more extensive examination of the diagnostic procedures developed by A. R. Luria and his associates may be a good choice. To begin with, it incorporates a great deal of

factual knowledge about the brain obtained in the school
of neuropsychology established by Luria. It is also of
considerable interest per se - the fact that a great many
neuropsychologists from all over the world keep coming to
learn more about these methods of diagnostics speaks for
itself. Beyond this, the Luria battery of tests may give,
as a result of some analysis, some insight into the very
philosophy of understanding the brain-behavior relations
which has been developed by several generations of Soviet
psychologists, starting with Vygotskii. It is, in a sense,
a scientific credo converted into the form of a practical,
clinical tool, in which the credo has been crystallized.

     In fact, the experimental techniques devised by Luria
for approaching focal brain lesions have never been
published in the form of an explicit and compact manual,
although a careful reader can extract them from Higher
Cortical Functions in Man (1966), The Working Brain (1973),
and numerous other books by A. R. Luria translated in the
USA. In these writings, however, the experimental
techniques themselves are incorporated into a more theoretical context, which provides rationale and justification
for them. This circumstance, the fact that an extremely
interesting and widely acknowledged method of focal brain
lesion diagnostics has never been presented overtly in a
compact way, makes worthwhile doing it here.

     Following is an abbreviated description of the test
battery designed (or rather brought together) by Luria.
It does not cover all the experimental procedures used in
this school of neuropsychology for local diagnostic purposes. After all, the present paper is not supposed to be
a manual. Rather it is an attempt to give an idea of a
certain experimental approach, and to provide the basis for
analysis of the philosophy that underlies it.

     The whole battery can be subdivided into parts, which
deal with "faculties" of behavior. Each of these parts is
abbreviated in the present description. The group of
tests pertaining to concept-formation and what may be
vaguely called "abstract thinking" has been completely
deleted, except for numeric operations. Also those tests
which are usually included in neurological examinations
were completely deleted. The descriptions of the tests
are deleted in cases where the names of the tests are

sufficient to give an idea about the actual procedures
implied.

Some of the data and techniques discussed below were
obtained (or devised) by Luria himself, some of them by
other authors. So, instead of giving references for all the
findings and techniques mentioned in this paper, there will
be given a list of selected writings by Luria, where he
traces the history of every finding he utilizes and gives
tribute to its author. It will enable an interested reader
to find out what the original sources of information and
ideas used by Luria in his approach were, from his own
point of view.

I. MOTOR PROCESSES

1. Posture Praxis

The patient must imitate and carry out under verbal
instructions various postures of his hands.

Possible implications:

A. Nonsystematic difficulties in performance
indicate impairment of the kinesthetic control
of movements (involvement of postcentral area of
the motor projective zone, contralateral side);

B. "Mirror effects" with corrections available
indicate the impairment of visual-spatial
coordination (involvement of left parieto-
temporal area);

C. Perseverations and/or "mirror effects" without
corrections indicate involvement of prefrontal
areas.

This test is reported to be most sensitive for case (A)

2. Dynamic Praxis

Imitating and performing kinetic sequences upon verbal
instruction, like touching the thumb with the other fingers
sequentially, or striking a surface with the fingers in the
following order: 1, 2, 3; 1, 2, 3, 4, 5...

A possible implication in the case of performance discrepancies is that the precentral motor area of the contralateral side is affected by the lesion.

3. Spatial Organization of Movements

The patient must imitate various asymmetric arm postures, while demands on the subtle kinesthetic aspect of the movements are minimal.

Possible Implications:

A. Nonsystematic and correctible "mirror" errors indicate parieto-temporo-occipital areas being affected by the lesion (no specification can be made as to the lateralization);

B. Perseverations and noncorrectible "mirror" errors indicate a prefrontal lesion.

The test is reported to be most sensitive for case (A).

3a. Hedd Test

A modification of test 3. It is reported to be most sensitive for case (3B).

4. Reciprocal Coordinations (Ozeretskii Test)

The test consists of reciprocal change in the hand postures.

Possible implications:

A. A delay of one hand's performance may indicate a contralateral premotor area lesion;

B. Total inability to perform the test with both hands, while being able to do it with each hand separately, indicates that the anterior portions of the corpus callosum are affected by the lesion.

II. THE SEQUENTIAL ORGANIZATION OF ACTIONS

1. Breaking a Stereotypic Sequence

The patient is instructed to respond in definite ways to two types of signals. Then the signals are presented in stereotypic sequence: A-B-A-B.... After that the stereotype is broken by the experimenter: A-B-A-B-A-B-B-B-A-B-A-A....

Possible implications:

If the patient continues to respond in a stereotypic way after the actual sequence of instructions has been changed, it may indicate that prefrontal areas are affected by the lesion. This suggestion will be valid only if there is evidence that the patient remembers the actual instruction.

2. Introduction of a "Provoking Signal"

The patient is instructed to lift his left arm in response to one auditory signal, and the right arm in response to two auditory signals.

Possible implications:

If the patient's reactions imitate the stimulus properties (the arm is lifted twice, when two auditory signals are presented, and once, when one signal is presented), it strongly indicates that the prefrontal areas are affected by the lesion.

This test is more sensitive to prefrontal lesions than the previous one.

2a. Conflict Reactions

The patient is instructed to lift a fist when the experimenter lifts a finger, and vice versa.

Implications are the same as in the previous test. This variant of the test is much more sensitive than test 2.

The tests 1, 2, 2a do not provide a very good
differentiation between the prefrontal convexital and
fronto-basal areas, although there is some evidence that
in the latter case the errors are more correctible.

3. Drawing Graphic Sequences

The patient is instructed to draw sequences of simple
geometric figures according to verbal instructions. The
test can be performed like test 1, or without any regularity
of the figure order. In the former case the implications
will be as in test 1.

Otherwise, there may be the following implications:

A. Hyperkinesis-like perseverations will indicate
    that the medial (deep) premotor areas are
    affected by the lesion;

B. Contamination-type perseverations indicate
    that the prefrontal areas are affected by
    the lesion.

There is some preliminary evidence, although not yet
validated, that the different types of (B) refer differentially to convexital prefrontal, medio-basal and posterior-
frontal areas. It is almost impossible to differentiate
between these areas in any other way.

4. Performance of "Reversed" Sequences

The patient is instructed to perform memorized
sequences in a reversed way, e.g., naming the months in
reverse, starting with December.

Possible implications:

Difficulties in performing the test and the tendency
to return to the "standard" sequence, may indicate that the
prefrontal areas are affected by the lesion.

III. VISUAL PERCEPTION

1. <u>Recognition and Naming of Pictures of Objects</u>

Possible implications (all of them still leave open
the possibility of aphasic deficits being involved
instead of or in addition to the visual perception
difficulties proper. That is why the data obtained
with this test should be evaluated together with
the speech function data):

A. Giving the name of the class of objects instead
of the object itself would indicate that the
right occipito-parietal areas are affected
by the lesion;

B. Misnaming or misrecognizing the object on the
basis of an elementary sensory property
(usually, color) may have the same implications as (A), or may indicate that the
prefrontal areas are affected by the lesion;

C. Misnaming or misrecognizing the object on
the basis of the shape properties that are
common to the object presented and the object
actually named, would indicate that the left
occipito-parietal areas are affected by the
lesion. It may also indicate, although with
a lower probability, that the prefrontal areas
are involved.

2. <u>Recognition and Naming of Contour Pictures</u>

This test should be administered after test 1.

Possible implications:

If the level of performance of this test is worse
than that of test 1, this would indicate that the
left occipito-parietal area is affected by the
lesion.

2a. <u>Recognition of Contour Pictures with "Noise"</u>

Contour pictures crossed over with lines are presented
to the subject.

2b. Poppelreuter Test

Overlapping contour pictures are presented to the subject for recognition and naming.

Tests 2a and 2b are more sensitive variants of test 2, with the same implications. Test 2b is more sensitive than test 2a.

3. Face Recognition

The subject is presented with a series of photographs, which he must sort into groups representing the same person.

Possible implications:

Failure to perform this task indicates that the right occipito-parietal area is affected by the lesion.

4. Asymmetric Figure Identification

The subject is presented with a set of asymmetric figures and a control one, which has to be identified in the set properly.

Possible implications:

The failure to perform the task indicates that the parieto-occipital areas are affected by the lesion (most probably the left one, although the right one may respond to the test too).

4a.

The same test can be administered in the form of copying asymmetric figures, with the same implications.

5. Asymmetric Symbolic Pattern Differentiation

The subject is instructed to tell the time on a schematic clock which lacks numbers; or choose the correct geographic map out of two, where one is mirror-inverted; or do the same task with letters or numbers.

Possible implications:

If the patient is unable to differentiate between the proper and inverted patterns, it indicates that the left parieto-occipital area is affected by the lesion.

IV. NUMERIC OPERATIONS

1. Serial Subtraction

The patient is instructed to serially subtract 7 from 100 (orally): (100 - 7) -7...

Possible implications:

A. Stereotypic performance (e.g., 100 ... 93 ... 83 ... 73 ...) would indicate frontal lobes being affected by the lesion;

B. Difficulties with the number placement on the natural axis (right-left confusions), e.g., 100... 93 ... 84 ... 73 ...) would indicate that the left parieto-occipital areas are affected by the lesion;

C. Failure to accomplish the operation of adjusting the first digit of the number (e.g., 100 ... 93 ... 96 ... 89 ... 82 ... 85 ...) would indicate nonspecific memory deficits of diencephalic nature.

1a.

Essentially the same test can be administered as a series of separate mathematical operations, with the same implications.

2. Evaluation of Numbers

The subject is instructed to decide which of the two numbers presented is bigger.

Possible implications:

A. If judgments are made by the subject on the basis of individual numerals rather than on the basis of the numbers' order structure (e.g., 19>32), this would indicate that the left parieto-occipital areas or (less probably) prefrontal areas are affected by the lesion;

B. Nonsystematic errors would indicate that the
    prefrontal areas are involved.

V. AUDITORY NONVERBAL PERCEPTION

1. Comprehension of Tonal Relations

The patient is instructed to react with conditioned
responses towards two mutually reversed tone patterns, e.g.,
    versus   or sequences of patterns like:
and   versus   and

Possible implications:

Inability to perform the discrimination tasks may
indicate that the nuclear part of the temporal
lobe (most probably, right) is affected by the
lesion. This implication is valid only if
similar differentiations are possible in other
sensory modalities (visual and tactile). Then
it would mean that it is not a matter of nonspecific memory disturbances

                        1a.

The patient is instructed to reproduce patterns of the
above type.

Possible implications:

As above; or left motor lower areas; or postcentral zone lower areas, are affected by the
lesion.

2. Rythmical Pattern Evaluation

The patient is presented with a rythmical structure
several times, e.g., ||| '' (where | means a loud knock;
' means a soft one) with the instructions to tell how many
knocks, or how many loud and how many soft knocks there
were in the pattern.

Possible implications:

Inability to perform this task would indicate that

the nuclear zone of the left or right temporal
lobe is affected by the lesion.

A. If an increase of the pattern presentation
    speed (with 1.5 - 2 sec intervals between
    the patterns) facilitates the subject's
    task performance, then it would indicate that
    the left temporal lobe is involved;

B. If vice versa, then the right temporal lobe
    should be suspected.

    This differentiation, however, is not of
    great reliability.

3. Rythmical Pattern Reproduction Following a Sample
         Versus Following Verbal Instruction

The patient is instructed to reproduce rythmical
patterns according to auditory samples, and according to
verbal instructions as in test 2.

Possible implications:

Difficulties in performing these tasks may
indicate that nuclear areas of the temporal lobes
or premotor and/or frontal areas are affected by
the lesion.

If the performance in response to the auditory sample
is better than that in response to the verbal instructions, it may indicate that premotor or frontal areas
are affected by the lesion. If vice versa, then the
temporal lobes should be suspected.

VI. SPEECH COMPREHENSION

1. Sensory Ability for Phonemic Differentiation

The patient is instructed to reproduce and to recognize
(among the graphemes) pairs of sounds:

a. disjunctive: [m] - [r] ; [p] - [s] ; [b] - [n]

b. oppositional or correlating: [b] - [p] ; [d] - [t];
    [k] - [g]

c. sequences of three sounds: [a]- [o] - [u] ;
[b] - [r] - [k] ; [m] - [s] - [d].

Possible implications:

Inability to make the above differentiations
indicates:

A. Sensory aphasic difficulties - upper-posterior
part of the left temporal area is affected
by the lesion;

B. Afferent motor aphasic difficulties - lower
parts of the left postcentral area are
affected by the lesion.

2.   Kinesthetic Aspect of Phonemic Differentiation

The patient is instructed to reproduce and recognize
pairs of sounds which differ acoustically but have very
close articulatory patterns, e.g., [b] - [m]; [d] - [n].

Possible implications:

A. A relatively poorer performance on this test
than on 1a and 1c would indicate afferent
motor aphasia;

B. If otherwise, it would indicate sensory
aphasia.

3.   Reproduction of Syllable Sequences

The patient is instructed to repeat sequences of
syllables with a fixed consonant and a varying vowel, e.g.,
[bi] - [ba] - [bo], and to switch from one sequence to
another: [bi] - [ba] - [bo] ➡ [ba] - [bo] - [ba] ➡
[bo] - [bi] - [ba].

Possible implications:

Inability to perform this task may indicate
efferent motor aphasic difficulties - lower
parts of the left precentral and/or premotor
areas being affected by the lesion. This

judgment is valid only if the performance on
test 3 is poorer than that on tests 1 and 2.

4. Common Word Comprehension

a. The patient is instructed to select the pictures
(or objects) which correspond to the words named to him.

b. The patient is instructed to perform this task
when a series of two or three words is presented to him
simultaneously (sensitized variant).

c. The patient is instructed to perform this task
when the words presented are close phonetically (literally
or verbally).

Possible implications:

Inability to perform these tasks may indicate sensory
aphasic or acoustico-mnestic aphasic difficulties.
(Brodmann areas 21, 37)

A. Literal paraphasias underlying the errors
   of selection may support the first hypothesis;

B. Verbal paraphasias would support the second
   hypothesis.

5. Memorizing of Short Word and Phrase Sequences

The patient is instructed to reproduce short word
sequences (3 words) and two-component phrase sequences
(2-3 phrases), under the following conditions: (a)
immediately after presentation, and (b) after a 5-10
sec pause.

Possible implications:

A. If the performance in this test is poorer than
   in the previous test (object-naming), this
   may indicate acoustico-mnestic aphasic
   difficulties, the middle area of the left
   temporal lobe (Brodmann areas 21, 37) being
   affected by the lesion. Or it may imply that
   the medial part of the left temporal lobe is
   affected by the lesion.

B. Perseveratory performance of the task may
    indicate that the left fronto-temporal areas
    are affected by the lesion. This suggestion
    will be valid only if no perseverations are
    observed in nonverbal tests;

C. The possibility of modality nonspecific memory
    deficits (involvement of diencephalic structures)
    is left open. See tests VIII - 1, 2 below.

6. Comprehension of Logico - Grammatical Relations

a. The patient is instructed to give names to attribu-
tive constructions, e.g , "the father's brother (the
uncle)" versus "the brother's father (the father)";

b. He is instructed to demonstrate comprehension of
prepositions dealing with spatial and temporal relations
(before, under, etc.) by selecting a picture relevant to
the given construction (e.g., "a book under the table");
or by drawing a relevant picture; or by stating which of the
two alternative constructions is proper (e.g., "Tuesday comes
before Monday" or vice versa).

Possible implications:

Inability to accomplish these tasks indicates
semantic aphasic difficulties - the left temporo-
parieto-occipital areas are affected by the
lesion.

VII. EXPRESSIVE SPEECH

1. Nominative Speech

The patient is instructed to name the objects or
pictures presented to him.

Possible implications:

A. Literal paraphasias and inability to name
    the object after the first syllable of the
    proper word has been prompted to the patient
    may indicate sensory aphasic difficulties
    (upper posterior part of the left temporal
    lobe is affected by the lesion);

B. Verbal paraphasias and lack of improvement
    after the prompt may indicate acoustico-
    mnestic aphasic difficulties (Brodmann
    areas 21, 37 being involved);

C. Immediate effect of the prompt may indicate
    (although not with great reliability)
    amnestic aphasic difficulties - the left
    parieto-occipital area is involved.

2. Dialogic Speech

This is an exploratory communication with the patient
rather than a standardizable test. The experimenter asks
the patient questions about current events.

Possible implications:

A. Echolalic responses would strongly suggest
    that the convexital and/or basal areas of
    the prefrontal lobes are affected by the
    lesion (provided that no discrepancies had
    been found in the previous speech-related
    tests. Otherwise the left fronto-temporal
    area is also a possibility);

B. "Telegraphic style," lack of predicative
    components; and/or perseverations (provided
    that they were not observed in nonspeech
    tests), would indicate that the lower parts
    of the left premotor area are affected by
    the lesion;

C. Lack of nominative components and "over-
    predicated" speech, as well as verbal
    paraphasias, would indicate acoustico-
    mnestic difficulties (Brodmann areas 21,
    37 being involved).

Other possible types of discrepancies and their implications are not described here. They are covered by the above-
described speech-related tests, or in the following part,
dealing with memory.

3. Reproduction of Short Stories

The test is administered as immediate reproduction, following oral presentation of the story. Implications as for test 2. Modifications of the same test will be discussed below (VIII-3), with some other possible implications.

3a. An Oral Composition on a Well-Known Topic

(e.g., describing what the job of a cabdriver consists of).

Implications as in the previous test.

4. Accomplishing Syntactic Constructions

The patient must fill in the blank in a sentence with a syntactic unit, e.g., "The airplane crashed (although) the engine was in good shape."

Possible implications:

The test is most sensitive towards semantic-aphasic difficulties (temporo-parieto-occipital parts of the left hemisphere being affected). But it may also respond to prefrontal lesions.

VIII.   MEMORY PROCESSES

1. Immediate Recognition and Recall

The patient is presented with a series of 3-4 pictures of objects or geometric figures, with the instruction to memorize them. The stimuli are presented for 5-7 sec. Immediately after the presentation, the patient must (a) name or reproduce the stimuli; (b) select them from a larger set of stimuli.

The same experiment should be administered in the auditory modality (series of rythms or sounds); verbal mode (series of words); and kinesthetic modality (series of hand postures).

Possible implications:

A. Failure to perform the task in all the
    modalities to the same extent, would indicate
    that the diencephalic structures are affected
    by the lesion;

B. Failure to perform the task in one modality
    to as great an extent as in others, would
    indicate that the corresponding gnostic
    area is affected by the lesion.

Variant (B) is usually accompanied by perceptual
deficits in the corresponding modality (according to the
above described perceptual tests). Then the evaluation of
the relative extent of memory versus immediate perception
deficits in the given modality, may indicate how deep (or
how convexital) the lesion is.

2. Delayed Recognition and Recall

The test is similar to the previous one, with the
following modifications:

a. The patient must respond after a pause of 10 sec to 10
    min (the longer the interval, the more sensitive the
    experiment);

b. After a pause of 10 sec to 10 min filled with
    heterogeneous interference, e.g., numeric operations;

c. After homogeneous interference: the task to memorize
    another similar sequence of stimuli.

    Possible implications are as in test 1. However,
    test 2 is more sensitive towards memory deficits,
    modality-nonspecific ones, in particular. The
    sensitivity towards lesions increases from
    (a) to (c).

3. Reproduction of Short Stories

This test should be administered in four ways, as
tests 1, 2a, 2b, 2c (in this case, another story serves as
homogeneous interference). The sensitivity of the variants
increases from 1 to 2c.

Apart from the above discussed aphasic possibilities,
there are the following possible implications:

A. Omitting parts of the story; tendency to recall
    it in overgeneralized way (with logistic
    compensation); failure to recollect the
    mere fact of the first story presentation in
    case 3c, would indicate that the hypophysis
    is affected by the lesion; or that a unilateral
    hippocampal lesion is present;

B. Contaminations in case 3c and arbitrary
    replacements of the original story fragments
    by irrelevant, although plausible ones,
    would indicate a bilateral hippocampal
    lesion, or any other massive lesion affecting
    the Papez circuit (e.g., mammillary bodies);

C. Nonrestricted confabulations with the general
    framework of the story still being preserved,
    would indicate that the higher stem is
    affected by the lesion;

D. Verbal "field behavior" (following the chain
    of stereotypic or individual associations)
    leading away from the original topic, would
    indicate that prefrontal areas are affected by
    the lesion. Verbal and topic perseverations
    would have the same implications.

Besides the "pure" cases mentioned above, there are
several types of very frequently observed and more or less
distinct mixed cases.

Although it would be very difficult to introduce
quantitative scoring in this test, its heuristic value for
singling out the level of nonspecific systems affected by
the lesion (A - C), and the differentiation of memory
deficits from pseudo-anmestic prefrontal phenomena, is very
great.

For obvious reasons, judgments derived from this test
should be dependent on the testing of speech-processes, as
described above.

4. Memory Learning Curve

A series of 10 one-syllable words is presented to the patient, with the instruction to reproduce it. After the task is fulfilled, the procedure recurs, and so on, until the subject is able to reproduce the whole series. For a normal subject it usually takes 4-5 trials.

Possible implications:

A. A "rigid" learning curve (9-10 trials, with 8 words as the limit) with small overlapping of the words reproduced in consecutive trials, would indicate that diencephalic or left temporo-medial areas are affected by the lesion;

B. A "Plato"-type curve (which approaches the amount of 5-6 words rapidly without subsequent growth) with great overlapping of the words reproduced in consecutive trials, would indicate that prefrontal or medio-basal areas are affected by the lesion.

The above described approach to the diagnostics of focal brain lesions may cause considerable dissatisfaction in an American psychologist, since it does not meet some basic methodological requirements.

Nevertheless, it passes the ultimate pragmatic test perfectly well; maybe better than any other existing test battery of this type. The correlation between the prediction as to the locus of a lesion made on the basis of the above techniques and the reports about the lesion which follow the actual neurosurgical procedure or post-mortem examination, is extremely high. It is even more striking provided that (as the reader might have already noticed) the neuropsychological statements are being made in fairly precise terms; it is not just deciding whether the lesion is "anterior" versus "posterior," "cortical" versus "subcortical," or "left" versus "right."

These circumstances may encourage certain American neuropsychologists to try to elaborate the above described collection of techniques to make it meet some basic methodological requirements. Let us try to make a sketch of the problems which ought to be overcome in order to achieve this goal.

To begin with, the experimental procedures involved are not completely standardized. However, this can be done easily.

A much more complicated problem would be that of designing nonambiguous criteria of clustering different types of errors which are potentially possible in the given test performance. The problem will arise then of measuring (scoring) the amount of a given particular type of error. It can be done in a fairly obvious way with some tests, but with others it may create a real problem. So, more or less arbitrary measure will have to be postulated in the beginning, with subsequent refinement in the course of the test validation.

All the above described difficulties can be overcome in principle and the battery can be converted into a standardized form. If so, considerable redundancy of the battery will become obvious. This is due to the fact that double procedure is involved in the testing: (a) if the items of each test are evaluated on a pass-fail basis, the experimenter obtains from each test very little information as to the type of lesion, so a large (if not the whole) part of the battery will have to be involved to obtain the necessary information; (b) on the other hand, if the above described analysis of qualitative types of errors provided by the tests is used, then the information provided by each separate test will be much greater, and a relatively small part of the battery may be sufficient to accomplish the evaluation procedure. So it would be up to the experimenter to either reduce the resolving capacity of each test and to utilize many of them in a diagnostic procedure; or to utilize the full resolving capacity of each test while applying a relatively small subset of them.

As the reader may have realized, the actual procedure for applying the battery is not that of obtaining a "profile" across all the tests, and then relating certain profiles to certain statements as to localization of disease but rather a sequential procedure of going through a "logical tree."

The above given sketch of the Luria battery of tests

was described here in the form of its "decomposition"; the
relations between separate tests in the process of evaluation have not been emphasized.

Ideally speaking, in its composed form the battery can
be viewed as a logical tree with a very wide "branching" in
the beginning and a relatively short termination of each
sequence of branches, leading to a precise statement with
very high reliability. This allows one to generate an
"algorithmic" form of the battery. A psychologist with
the ambition to do so will have to confront the problem of
assigning empirical approximations of two types of
conditional probabilities: probabilities of a given type of
lesion, provided a given outcome of a given test arises,
(L_i/T_{jn}), and probabilities of a given outcome of a given
test, provided there is a given type of lesion P (T_{jn}/L_i).
The first type of probabilities, actually, are quantitative
evaluations of what had been listed in the sketch of the
battery as "possible implications." They pertain to
deriving hypotheses as to the locus of the lesion. The
second type of probabilities would serve as the means of
selecting the most informative procedures of testing the
hypothesis once it has emerged. The whole problem is a
fairly complicated one, if one were to go through the
sequential steps of evaluation, and we will not discuss it
here.

And, finally, it is quite obvious that introduction of
all the quantitative measures described will need validation
with a local brain damage population, where refined instru-
mental analysis, like brain screening, and the results of
neurosurgical intervention would serve as validity criteria.

In fact, without introducing standard scores and
reliability measures for each local statement, the diagnostic techniques described are used in the neuropsychological
laboratory at Burdenko Institute in Moscow with fairly high
precision, and just in the way of a "follow-the-logical-tree"
procedure. It means that on an intuitive level, all these
variables are "computed" in the head of an experienced
researcher - as often happens in clinical reality.

There are several circumstances to account for the
peculiar form of the above sketched test battery, which is
so different from most of those used by American
psychologists. It may be of some interest to screen them.

There has been a long-term bias in Soviet psychology against introducing quantitative parameters into behavioral and social sciences in general. The lack of quantitative methods is such an obvious shortcoming that there is no need to dwell upon it. However, in the particular case under discussion, this weakness is probably a sacrifice in order to preserve what has given the battery strong advantages over many other neuropsychological test batteries.

To begin with, Luria has never viewed his test battery simply as a pragmatic diagnostic technique, where the only thing that counted was high correlations between certain experimental findings and certain lesion loci, no matter whether the reasons for these correlations were known or not. Quite the contrary, the battery has been developed as a consequence of the understanding of relations between the operational structure of functions and constellations of the areas of the brain. This circumstance by itself explains why the battery could not possibly have taken the form of a "profile-drawing-type" test battery, instead of becoming a "logical-tree" procedure.

Another significant consequence of the fact that the battery was developed by theoretical considerations, rather than pragmatic ones, is the fact that those who designed it did not want to sacrifice phenomenology, in order to make the rough data more easily describable in quantitative terms. As demonstrated above, it is not "passing or failing" the test that is the most important cue for deriving a local hypothesis, but the particular type of error once the failure has been observed. Such an approach greatly enriches the information about the functional structure of behavioral discrepancies observed, but it also complicates the introduction of quantitative parameters. The question is, what sacrifice is a greater trade-off: clear-cut methodology or phenomenological richness? Probably what would be ideal from the point of view of an American psychologist desiring to elaborate Luria's test battery is to combine the two requirements: reasonable methodology and phenomenological richness.

The fact that the only neuropsychological test battery existing in the USSR is based on sophisticated brain-behavior relations theory, while some of the many ones existing in the USA are not, reflects a basic difference between the status of psychology in these two countries. While in the USA clinical psychology (including clinical neuropsychology) long ago obtained the status of an independent, applied area, in the USSR it is still a semi-acknowledged area of psychology as contrasted with basic research. There are no educational programs designed for predominantly clinical training. As a result, those few people who have chosen to deal with clinical issues, still do so as a byproduct of their research in basic psychology, and with a "cause-consequence" approach. The few attempts at clinical applications existing in the USSR are strongly influenced by certain theoretical assumptions and aspirations, with measurement itself being a secondary concern. These theoretical assumptions may have either good or bad effects. In the case of the clinical approach by A. R. Luria, the effect is presumably mostly good. However, it is not always so in many other instances.

Such a situation leads to the fact that although some of the clinical applications of psychology are excellent in Russia, the variety of approaches is limited and the total outcome in terms of serving human needs is negligible.

On the other hand, American clinical psychology, with its main preoccupation with providing immediate practical results in terms of community service and great variety of approaches, sometimes ceases to be regulated by theoretical conceptualizations. It follows its own laws of a purely applied branch of psychology. This means that many significant correlations among a great number of things have been obtained, but the clinicians do not know what they mean and sometimes do not even care to know, as long as the tests work. As far as purely pragmatic goals are concerned, it is very often a success, and the rewards are great. But the lack of interactions between psychometrics and brain-behavior theory is sometimes obvious.

There is another aspect of the Luria test battery which may be of some interest from the theoretical point of view.

It can be easily recognized that the tests constituting the battery are not measuring "factors" of information processing. This follows from the mere fact that each test is not evaluated on the dichotomous basis of "pass-fail."

On the contrary, it can lead to several qualitative types of errors. Each of the types can consequently be scored in terms of its severity. So, the possible variants of performing the given test can be described only in a multidimensional space. If the tests were of "factor-measuring" nature, one would expect them to be describable in unidimensional spaces, on the axis "pass-fail," with the severity of failure being scored.

Again, it is to a great extent the consequence of certain theoretical presumptions. Vygotskii, and later Luria, Leont'ev, Anokhin, introduced the concept of "the functional system" as a neurophysiological substrate of a given type of activity. The notion is as vague as any other psycholog-ical notion at this level of generalization, but it has certain implications. "A functional system" is a constel-lation of brain structures which becomes involved in subserving a given type of activity following its semantic structure, as determined by the cultural experience of the particular person. The cultural determination of the function-structures and their relations to the brain is the central point of the approach. Furthermore, the same logic is applied not only to certain types of activity, but to their basic constituents which can be viewed as "factors." The brain is viewed as a body which originally is to a great extent semantically indifferent (obviously, except for primary projection zones).

This can be demonstrated by the following example. A symbolic - nonsymbolic dichotomy in the distribution of hemispheric "responsibilities" is known for the adult brain. It not only includes the fact that speech is connected with the dominant hemisphere, but also indicates that certain types of visual and visual-spatial perception are more closely identified with the left hemisphere and others with the right one. For instance, perception of meaningful visual stimuli is affected when the left hemisphere is damaged, and the more schematic the meaning-ful figure is, the more it is connected with the left occipito-temporo-parietal areas. Contour figure recognition is known to be particularly impaired if the lesion is in the left hemisphere. On the other hand, those visual stimuli which are less easily described in terms of a discrete alphabet of features are reported to be misperceived when right hemisphere lesions are involved.

Thus, it is known that face recognition is impaired almost exclusively when the right temporal lobe is damaged. Interestingly enough, face recognition appeared to be an unsolvable problem in perceptronics, which may indicate that this type of visual discrimination is the least analyzable in terms of discrete descriptive systems.

If we turn to visual-spatial discrimination problems, the same dichotomy is observed. While immediate orientation in space and body-scheme "resides" in the right hemisphere (to be more accurate, is impaired when the lesions affect a right hemisphere), visual-spatial discrimination involving symbolic elements (map, clock, schematic contour asymmetric patterns) is impaired if the left hemisphere lesion is observed.

The picture of auditory perception in adults represents a strikingly similar dichotomy. Thus, music-pattern discrimination was found to be impaired if the right temporal lobe is damaged, except in professional musicians, i.e., those people who are used to perceive music in terms of a symbolic, discrete alphabet.

Another observation reported a peculiar type of writing disturbance in right temporal patients: omitting of vowels. It has been suggested by many linguists that the meanings (paradigmatic aspect of the word) are carried predominantly by consonants (this can also be traced in ancient languages, e.g., Hebrew).

All these data indicate that the left-right dichotomy is more than an explicit language versus non-language functional dichotomy. Rather it is a dichotomy between those types of information processing which are processed in terms of discrete schematized alphabets of any nature (including language per se), and those which are of more diffuse, natural origin.

The notion of culturally determined strategies and types of information processing versus natural ones is not new for psychology. This opposition apparently fits the hemispheric dichotomy very well. If so, can we believe that hemispheric dichotomy is predetermined by the "original design of the brain? Or is it rather a function of the developmental process?

If the latter assumption is true, then it means that the "alphabet-type" information processing is simply not there in little children, and the notion of symbolic-nonsymbolic dichotomy cannot be applied to the child's information processing at its very early stages.

There is a gap between developmental histories of natural versus symbolic types of information processing. The latter develop with a delay, since they are dependent on language and also must have a natural prerequisite in their acquisition. It means that hemispheric lateral-ization follows the cognitive growth of a child. The more symbolic-type information processing he acquires and the more refined it becomes, the more the hemispheric asymmetry is expressed.

Apparently, the property of information processing being symbolic versus natural meets the requirements of what can be treated as a factor in the adult behavior observa-tions. It appears, however, that it is not inherent in the brain from birth. Instead, it is a function of cultural growth. It has been demonstrated by numerous experimental studies, which we will not list here.

The notion that such factors cannot be viewed as a list of basic features of information processing which remains stable and unchangeable throughout the course of development, nevertheless leaves the question open, whether it is reasonable to apply "factor" philosophy to a given age sample and cultural background. For example, can it be applied to the adult population of Western culture where, indeed, neuropsychological observations demonstrate very strong invariants across the subjects in terms of the relations between the locus of the lesion and the functional impairments observed?

So, it may be a question of considerable interest, whether the "nonfactorial" approach to the local brain lesion diagnostics developed by A. R. Luria can have a reasonable "factorial" interpretation. Essentially, it is a question of whether "factorial" philosophy can be heuristic in the neuropsychological context. I suspect that A. R. Luria's answer to this question would be a positive "no." I guess that mine would be "no," too. But it is still a question - a question of what should our modifications of the concept "factor" be, if we want to apply it to brain-behavior relations as opposed to applying it to behavior itself, and what might the possible outcome of such an effort be.

ACKNOWLEDGMENTS

I thank Dr. R. Karrer and Dr. J. Wertch for their valuable suggestions and help in the preparation of this paper.

BIBLIOGRAPHY

LURIA, A. R. (1964). Neuropsychology in the diagnostics of brain damage. Cortex, No. 1.

LURIA, A. R. (1965). Neuropsychological analysis of focal brain lesions. In: B. B. Wolman, ed. Handbook of Clinical Psychology. New York, McGraw-Hill.

LURIA, A. R. (1965). Aspects of aphasia. J. Neurolog. Sciences, No. 2.

LURIA, A. R. (1965). L. S. Vygotskii and the problem of localization of functions. Neuropsychologia, No. 5.

LURIA, A. R. (1966). Higher Cortical Functions in Man. New York, Basic Books.

LURIA, A. R. (1966). Human Brain and Psychological Processes. New York, Harper & Row.

LURIA, A. R. (1969). The frontal syndrome. In: P. J. Vinken and G. W. Bruyn, eds. Handbook of Clinical Neurology, Vol. 2. Amsterdam, North-Holland Publ. Co.

LURIA, A. R. (1970). Traumatic Aphasia. The Hague, Mouton & Co.

LURIA, A. R. (1973). The Working Brain. New York, Basic Books, Inc.

LURIA (LURIYA), A. R. (1974). Neiropsikhologiya pamyati. Narusheniya pamyati pri lokal'nykh porazheniyakh mozga. I (Neuropsychology of Memory. Memory Disorders in Local Brain Lesions. Part I). Pedagogika, Moscow, 312 pp.

LURIA (LURIYA), A. R., AND E. Yu. ARTEM'EVA (1970). O dvukh
    putyakh dostizheniya dostovernosti psikhologicheskogo
    issledovaniya (On two ways of achieving reliability in
    psychological studies). Voprosy psikhologii (Problems
    of Psychology) No. 3: 105-112.

LURIA (LURIYA), A. R., AND E. D. KHOMSKAYA, eds. (1966).
    Lobnye doli i regulyatsiya psikhicheskikh protsessov
    (The Frontal Lobes and the Regulation of Mental
    Processes). Izd-vo MGU (Moscow State University
    Press), Moscow.

INTELLIGENCE, SOVIET DIALECTICS AND AMERICAN PSYCHOMETRICS;

IMPLICATIONS FOR THE EVALUATION OF LEARNING DISABILITIES

Robert H. Wozniak

Institute of Child Development
University of Minnesota
Minneapolis, Minnesota 55455

Until recently, American research in child psychology and special education has been widely influenced by a conception of intellectual process often referred to as the "psychometric perspective." Although considerable variation in the definition of intelligence has always existed among psychologists (Guilford, 1967; Terman, 1916; Spearman, 1927) sharing this perspective, a number of beliefs about the nature of intelligence are common to most psychometric views. Specifically, man is assumed to have some general ability to adapt to changing circumstances in his environment. This general ability to adapt is presumed to vary both within individuals over time and between individuals at any given point in their lives. Furthermore, this adaptive ability and its variations are assumed to be measurable and quantifiable; and individuals may then be at least roughly ordered along a purely quantitative continuum from those who adapt best to those who adapt most poorly. Lastly, it is commonly held that although the intellectual development of an individual is invariably influenced by the environmental circumstances in which he finds himself, individual variation in inheritance places differing limits on developmental potential and differentially conditions the rates with which individual intelligences develop.

For many reasons, this traditional psychometric perspective on human intellectual function and the intelligence tests around which it has developed have become a target of political, social, and scientific criticism (McClelland, 1973; Valett, 1972; Williams, 1973). The

bases of such criticism have been many and varied, ranging
from a social repugnance to the notion of a progression in
society toward an intellectual meritocracy to well-grounded
scientific appeals for the development of a theory of intelligence which might provide a better basis for psycho-
educational diagnosis.   Such a theory of intelligence might
give educators a tool to generate not a global and at best
moderately useful IQ score but a functional analysis of a
child's learning abilities and disabilities and specific
suggestions for using the child's abilities to overcome his
disabilities.

Criticisms of this type have prompted a number of developmental psychologists (cf., Riegel, 1973, for a series of
papers devoted to this topic) to examine conceptions of intellectual process alternative to that embodied in the
psychometric perspective.   One such alternative is that
which exists within Soviet psychology.   The Soviet view
stresses the fundamentally dialectical and socio-cultural
nature of intelligence and holds that these characteristics
are antithetical to both the philosophy and practice of
standardized psychometrics.   The purpose of this paper will
be to provide a brief description of the Soviet dialectical
and socio-cultural view of intelligence and to discuss the
consequences of this perspective for the theory of Soviet
psycho-educational diagnosis.

Intelligence and dialectics.   The form of the theory
of intelligence held by many Soviet psychologists is determined by specific assumptions about the nature of development.   These assumptions and their application to the analysis of an object or event in its physical and social context may be referred to as the "dialectical method"
(Wozniak, 1975a).   A primary principle of dialectics is
that everything exists in a process of constant alteration
and development.   An adequate understanding of the objects
and events of the real world can only be achieved within
the context of a developmental analysis.   For psychology
this implies that a theory of intelligence must be a theory
of intelligence in its development.   The psychologist must
attempt to understand the present organization (or disor-
ganization) of psychological processes in terms of its
developmental history.   A theory of intelligence should be
based on knowledge of the form of the organization of
psychological processes at different points of development

and of the reorganizations in these functional relationships which occur over time.

In addition to implying the necessity of an analysis
of objects and events in their development, the dialectical
method involves certain assumptions concerning the form of
development.   First, development is presumed to result
from the presence of internal tendencies in all objects
and events which are mutually incompatible but simultaneously presuppose one another (e.g., the necessity of an
organism to adapt to the constraints imposed upon it by
the environment while at the same time altering the environment so as to bring it into conformity with the organism's own internal structure).   It is the tension resulting from the contradictory yet mutually inclusive nature of opposite internal tendencies which provides the
impetus for development.   For psychology this suggests that
intelligence should be conceived as an active, organizing
force which directs the organism's interactions with the
environment and in so doing comes progressively to a more
adequate reflection of the structure of that environment.
Human intelligence, in other words, carries within itself
the motive force for its own self-development toward a
deeper understanding of reality.   Soviet psychologists view
this conception as incompatible with a view of intelligence
which characterizes it in terms of a fixed capacity.

Second, a dialectical analysis proceeds from the
assumption that development is formally both continuous
and discrete.   Real objects and events undergo gradual
quantitative change in a close relation to more sudden
qualitative shifts in organization.   A commonly cited example of such change is the physical state transition.
Continuous increase (or decrease) along a purely quantitative continuum (temperature) leads at certain points to
qualitative shifts in the state of a substance (e.g., water
changes into steam).   For psychology, the notion that development is both quantitative and qualitative and that
quantity and quality are intimately related suggests that
an understanding of the developing intelligence cannot be
based solely on a quantitative measurement of ability or
even on an analysis of the pattern of quantitative relationships among a set of independently measured abilities
(e.g., on an ability profile).   On the contrary, developing intelligence must first be understood in terms of the

systematic relations which obtain, at different periods of
development, among the various psychological functions.
The qualitative structure of intelligence and its altera-
tions over time must be considered as a whole. Only within
the framework of such a characterization of the total organizational structure of intelligence can quantitative
changes in intellectual functioning (e.g., an increase in
the information which an organism can bring to bear on the
organization of his action in a given situation) be ade-
quately conceptualized. It is worth noting that on this
issue Soviet psychology appears to be in fundamental agreement with other non-psychometrically oriented intelligence
theorists, most notably Piaget (1950).

Intelligence and socio-cultural interaction. In
addition to emphasizing the developmental nature of intelligence, Soviet theorists also stress the role played by
productive social activity in intellectual growth. In
their view, society, language, and culture have evolved
historically from group production. In turn, socio-cultural
and linguistic interaction provide man with tools to alter
his surroundings, thereby eliciting feedback which develops
his own intelligence. It was from this socio-cultural perspective that Vygotsky (cf., Leont'ev & Luria, 1968 for an
excellent, if brief, summary of Vygotsky's point of view)
developed a theory of cognitive development which has had
a major influence on contemporary psychological and educational practice in the Soviet Union.

Vygotsky stressed the critical role played by processes like language or mnemonic activity in cognitive
development. These processes, which he referred to as
"cultural mediators", are employed in and develop out of
the social interaction of adults with children. With
development, children internalize aspects of the structure
of such social interactions as a means of self-regulation
of their own higher mental processes (Vygotsky, 1962). In
other words, psychological functions which are at first
embedded in the child's external social activity, shared
with an adult (e.g., communicative speech), become the
individual internalized psychological processes of the
child (e.g., egocentric speech is internalized as the basis
for verbal thinking).

In addition to this socially developed character of

the "cultural mediators", Vygotsky also emphasized the re-
flective relationship which such mediators bear to reality.
The "cultural mediators", for Vygotsky, always represent
one or another aspect of the physical or social world.
Through the use of such representations, the child becomes
able on his own to introduce changes into external reality
which may in turn reflect back upon and develop his intelligence. By altering his environment, the child becomes
able to regulate his own behavior and control his own
psychological processes. He ceases to be completely dependent on the reality of the external situation.

   Dialectics, the socio-cultural perspective and psycho-
educational diagnosis. The impact of a dialectical, socio-
cultural theory of intelligence on Soviet child psychology
and special education is clearly exemplified in the area
of psycho-educational diagnosis. In evaluating a child
who is failing in his regular school work for placement in
a special program or in a special school for the mentally
retarded, Soviet psychologists (Vlasova & Pevzner, 1971)
argue for the use of a wide variety of medical, psychological, and educational observations. Although this advocacy
of a multi-faceted approach to evaluation and even the task
content of the evaluation itself is generally both traditional and similar to its typical American medical and
psychometric counterpart (Brožek, 1972), the form of the
observational procedure differs widely from the American
approach.

   First, both the task administration and the evaluation
of the child's performance are essentially clinical and
diagnostic rather than standardized and psychometric.
Second, and particularly when there is a question of dis-
criminating between children with learning problems ("de-
layed psychological development") and those with a form of
organic mental retardation, diagnostic tasks are administered in a multi-step process. Initially, the child is
asked to perform a task independently. Next he is asked
to perform the same or similar tasks while being provided
with a graded series of organizing assists from the examiner.
Finally, the child is once again asked to perform independently. Employing this format the diagnostician is able
to take into account not only the characteristics of the
child's initial approach to the task, but also his ability
to profit from the assistance provided in social inter-

action with an adult and to transfer these techniques to
subsequent independent performance. Third, at no point
does the Soviet diagnostician employ a normative, single-
administration psychometric instrument of the type common
in the United States and elsewhere (e.g., the Stanford-
Binet, WISC,* etc.). Since the 1930s, such tests have been
severely criticized and rejected in the Soviet literature.

Although a discussion of the complex series of political, economic, and scientific events leading to the rejection of standardized psychometrics in the USSR is clearly
beyond the scope of this paper (cf., Bauer, 1952; Wortis,
1950, for some discussion of these events), a brief summary
of current objections to Western-style standardized
testing will help to illustrate the close relationship between the relatively unusual format of Soviet diagnostic
evaluation and the guiding principles of a dialectical,
socio-cultural theory of intelligence.

The Soviet critique of standardized psychometrics.
Soviet psychologists are definitely not, as is occasionally
thought, opposed to all evaluation of intellectual performance. On the contrary, the structure of the Soviet system
of special schools necessitates decisions concerning student
placement (Vlasova & Pevzner, 1971); and this, in turn, requires such evaluation. Rather, the Soviet psycho-
educational literature indicates that it is the standardized, single administration, and, from the Soviet point of
view, overly quantified IQ test which is objectionable.

One source of this attitude, particularly that which
relates to the heavy reliance in psychometrics on quantification (specifically, the computation of an IQ), is
clearly political and philosophical, deriving from the
basic principles of Marxist thought. Thus, Zeigarnik
(1965) suggests that attempts to "measure" or quantify intelligence are based on the false notion that mental capacity is a fixed quantity and innate and that such development as occurs is merely linear, quantitative, and largely
predictable from earlier measurements.

From the dialectical Soviet perspective on intelligence, attempts at linear quantification of intelligence
lose sight of the potential for further development which
is inherent in human intellectual functioning. Rather than

*Wechsler Intelligence Scale for Children

indicating some inherent intellectual potential of the individual, standard psychometric methods estimate only the quantity of knowledge which an individual has already acquired. This static reliance on acquired knowledge is considered by Marxists to have serious political consequences. As Zeigarnik asserts: "Children of the higher strata of capitalist society, having been brought up in favorable conditions and having received a better education, reveal a wider range of knowledge in these (standardized psychometric) tests and are thereby enrolled in school with a higher educational standard than children of the less wealthy strata of society (p. 42)." In the Soviet Marxist view, in other words, psychometric tests are designed so as to perpetuate the class structure in capitalist society.

Soviet rejection of standardized psychometrics is not, however, by any means entirely based on political and philosophical objections. Soviet psychologists (Luria, 1961; Zeigarnik, 1965) point to a number of more purely scientific considerations which have led them to avoid the standardized psychometric approach. First, the heavy psychometric emphasis on the quantification of intellectual ability has traditionally resulted in the failure of psychometricians to emphasize the information which can be gained from an analysis of the qualitative aspects of poor performance. Variation in children's work methods, in the strategies which children bring to bear on the solution of problems, and in the attitudes toward tests and testers which the child brings to the testing situation are not and probably cannot be specifically taken into account in the computation of an IQ. Although a sensitive, experienced psychometrician can certainly observe these variations informally, the focus of the testing situation on specific types of response to specific, standardized questions reduces the extent to which the tester can afford to attend to these variables. Furthermore, in a psychometrically oriented system, a qualitative analysis of a child's poor performance may not be accorded the same "scientific" status by individuals in charge of placement decisions as is the computation of an IQ score.

Second, the relatively rigid nature of the standardized form of test item presentation in most psychometric evaluations drastically reduces the child's opportunity to employ his areas of developmental strength to compensate

for the areas in which he may be weak. Since compensatory
mechanisms of this type may be assumed to operate continuously in a child's adaptation to his home and classroom
environment, standardized psychometric evaluation is by its
nature unable to provide critical information concerning
a child's usual mode of adaptation. As a corollary weakness, the results of a standardized evaluation also typically fail to provide teachers with concrete applicable
guidelines for the organization of appropriate training
materials for the child.

Lastly, the care with which standardized tests are
constructed so as to minimize "contaminating" adult interaction and evaluate a child's "independent" performance
clearly ignores the critical fact that the child's intellectual development is a function of the internalization of
the form of social interactional processes, and that an
adequate evaluation of the child's level of development requires an evaluation of the child's ability to utilize
adult-provided information in problem solution.

Luria (1961), in his discussion of the social origins
of cognitive development, asks: "When we know that the
higher psychological processes, including intellectual
activity, have this complex developmental history and are
formed in the course of the child's speech-based social
relationships, can we continue to adhere to the former
static principles in assessing a child's abilities and in-
tellect? Can we continue to make confident judgments of a
child's intellectual development merely on whether he per-
forms a given task on his own with greater or lesser
success" (pages 40-41). In answer to his own question,
Luria suggests that a method of psychological evaluation
more in keeping with the central role of social processes
in intellectual development would receive a comparison
of initial independent performance with that under adult
assistance and then, particularly, with post-assistance
independent performance. This suggestion is similar to an
original notion of Vygotsky, the "zone of potential development" (Luria, 1961), involving measurement of the range
of potential development characteristic of a particular
child and manifest in his ability to profit from adult-
provided organizational cues.

The concept of "zone of potential development" has

recently become very influential in Soviet psycho-diagnosis, particularly with respect to the question of differentiating children with learning disabilities from MRs for the purposes of program assignment. For example, one major method (Luria, 1961; Egorova, 1969; Tsymbaliuk, 1973) of distinguishing among the three categories of functioning-- "normal," "learning disabled," and "mentally retarded"-- is to present the child with a task which requires that he supply missing organization to the materials. In such a situation, appropriately aged children who are functioning normally will be capable of providing some of the missing organization by themselves, but learning disabled and mentally retarded children will not. If, however, the same task is then presented again with increasing levels of adult organizational intervention (in which the adult provides the child with certain prompts in an attempt to help to organize the information in the task), the learning disabled child who may perform much more poorly than the normal child without such prompts, is capable of improving his performance virtually to a normal level through utilization of this additional organizing information. The mentally retarded, on the other hand, will generally be unable to take maximum advantage of the increased social organizational information to increase their performance.

Clearly, information of this type could not be gleaned from a single-administration, standardized IQ test. On the contrary, in fact, such single administration evaluation procedures are felt by Soviet theorists to provide a biased evaluation of a child's intellectual abilities, and, worse, as Zeigarnik (1965) has noted, the more pathological the subject's intellectual development (and often therefore the more important that the evaluation be accurate) the higher the likelihood that a typical psychometric test will lead to an inaccurate diagnosis.

Conclusion. It is hoped that from this relatively brief presentation, it may be seen that the Soviet view to psycho-educational diagnosis follows to a large extent from the particular form of the Soviet model of human intellectual development. This view of intellectual development, which is largely theoretical, is in turn conditioned by a set of more properly meta-theoretical or philosophical considerations. This meta-theory, embodied in the notion of dialectics, has not, traditionally, had much of an impact on the

construction of theory in American psychology. It is, however, the meta-theoretical perspective of other non-Soviet
theorists, most notably perhaps Piaget (Wozniak, 1975b).
Although there are important differences between the Soviet
view of intellectual development and Piaget's, in many
respects they are much more alike than either is similar to
the American psychometric tradition; and it is largely
through the impact of Piaget on American psychology that
American psychologists have begun to be forced to consider
conceptions of intelligence alternative to those embodied
in psychometrics. In this regard, a careful study of the
Soviet view, particularly, in terms of how it is similar
to and differs from that of Piaget, might be a worthwhile
endeavor for American psychologists looking for a more productive model of intelligence. Perhaps it will be possible
to evolve a synthesis of these approaches which will tran-
scend both.

BIBLIOGRAPHY

Bauer, R. A.   The New Man in Soviet Psychology.   Cambridge:
    Harvard University Press, 1952.

Brožek, J.   To test or not to test: Trends in the Soviet
    views.   Journal of the History of the Behavioral
    Sciences, 1972, 8, 243-248.

Egorova, T. V.   Analiz zritel'no vosprinimaemykh ob"ektov
    neuspevaiushchimi shkol'nikami mladshikh klassov
    (Analysis of visually perceived objects by failing
    students in the early grades).   Defektologiia, 1969
    (2), 29-37.

Guilford, J. P.   The Nature of Human Intelligence.   New
    York: McGraw-Hill, 1967.

Leont'ev, A. N. & Luria, A. R.   The psychological ideas of
    L. S. Vygotsky.   In B. B. Wolman (Ed.), Historical
    Roots of Contemporary Psychology.   New York: Harper
    & Row, 1968.

Luria, A. R.   Study of the abnormal child.   American
    Journal of Orthopsychiatry, 1961, 31, 1-16.

McClelland, D.   Testing for competence rather than for
    "intelligence."   American Psychologist, January 1973,
    1-14.

Piaget, J.   The Psychology of Intelligence.   London:
    Routledge & Kegan Paul Ltd., 1950.

Riegel, K. (Ed.).   An Epitaph for a Paradigm.   Human
    Development, 1973, 16, Whole No. 1-2.

Spearman, C.   The Nature of Intelligence and the Princi-
    ples of Cognition.   London: MacMillan and Co., Ltd.,
    1927.

Terman, L. M.   The Measurement of Intelligence.   New York:
    Houghton Mifflin Co., 1916.

Tsymbaliuk, A. N. Ponimanie siuzhetnoi kartiny v usloviiakh obuchaiushchego eksperimenta det'mi s zaderzhkoi razvitiia (Comprehension of a picture with a plot under conditions of a training experiment in children with retarded development). Defektologiia, 1973 (3), 25-32.

Valett, R. Developmental task analysis and psychoeducational programming. Journal of School Psychology, 1972, 10, 127-133.

Vlasova, T. A. & Pevzner, M. S. (Eds.). Deti s vremennymi zaderzhkami razvitiia. (Children with temporary retardation in development). Moscow: Pedagogika, 1971.

Vygotsky, L. S. Thought and Language. Cambridge: MIT Press, 1962.

Williams, R. A position paper on psychological testing of black people. Paper presented at the Annual Convention of the American Psychological Association, August, 1973, Montreal, Canada.

Wortis, J. Soviet Psychiatry. Baltimore: Williams and Wilkins Co., 1950.

Wozniak, R.H. A dialectical paradigm for psychological research: implications drawn from the history of psychology in the Soviet Union. Human Development, 1975a, 18, 18-34.

Wozniak, R.H. Dialecticism and structuralism: the philosophical foundations of Soviet psychology and Piagetian cognitive developmental theory. In K.F. Riegel and G.C. Rosenwald (Eds): Structure and Transformation: Developmental and Historical Aspects. New York: Wiley, 1975b.

Zeigarnik, B.V. The Pathology of Thinking. New York: Consultants Bureau, 1965.

A COMPARATIVE LOOK AT SOVIET PSYCHIATRY:

TRAINING, CONCEPTS, AND PRACTICE

Jimmie Holland

Dept. of Psychiatry, Montefiore Hospital
Albert Einstein School of Medicine
Bronx, New York

Under the Health Agreement signed in 1972 by the
Soviet Union and the United States, a collaborative
research project was undertaken by the Institute of
Psychiatry of the Academy of Medical Sciences in Moscow,
and the National Institute of Mental Health. The first
clinical phase of the work was done at the Institute in
Moscow during the academic year '72-'73. The project in
which I participated was a clinical study with Dr. Irina
Shakhmatova, aimed at understanding the Soviet classification of major mental illness. We attempted to develop a
system which incorporated the subtypes of schizophrenia
used by Soviet and American psychiatrists (2). Agreement
on clinical diagnosis of schizophrenia was necessary as
preparation for the second stage of the study in which
biological specimens from patients with schizophrenia
would be studied, as part of a collaborative research
program in biologic and genetic aspects of schizophrenia.
The biologic research, still in early planning stages,
continues to be developed. The impressions were gained
from observations made while working on the clinical
research study, and evaluating and treating patients on
one of the wards at Kaschenko Hospital. An overview of
major similarities and differences of Soviet psychiatry is
presented, with particular emphasis on education, concepts,
and clinical practice.

EDUCATION AND PSYCHIATRIC TRAINING

In considering psychiatric training, it is necessary
first to compare differences in both general and medical

133

education. Children in the USSR attend state-run nursery
schools from as early an age as 3 months, due to the fact
that most women have full-time jobs. The creches and nursery schools are well run, inexpensive and almost univer-
sally used by Russian mothers. Thus, children have a much
earlier and more intense group experience than American
children while growing up. The interesting effects upon
character development has been speculated upon by Bronfenbrenner (1), which have both positive and negative
aspects.

At age 7, the Soviet child begins Middle School. This
is equivalent to the 12 years of grammar and high school in
the United States. Children attend Middle School for 10
years from age 7 to 17 years (Fig. 1). In the last year of
Middle School, students compete intensively for the limited
places in universities and medical institutes. Acceptance
is based principally upon lengthy and difficult examinations.

The Medical Institute is a 6 year program beginning
after high school which includes both college and medical
school education, similar to the European model. A medical
student chooses one of the three possible curricula when he
enters: pediatrics, public health, or the therapeutic
faculty. Anyone choosing to do a general or specialized
medical practice will attend the therapeutic faculty. The
numbers of women continue to be over 50% in the Medical
Institute classes; among practicing physicians, women
account for 75% of the total. A graduate of the Medical
Institute is a fully qualified physician without further
examination or licensure. Many graduates take a one year
ordinatura in which they work as a physician in a specialty
hospital. Following apprenticeship in a psychiatric hospital, the physician may call himself a practicing psychiatrist, and accept a position in this specialty. Emphasis
is thus placed early in the young physician's career on
working as a specialist rather than upon obtaining broadly
based training as a general physician.

Only a small percentage, those who aspire to an
academic career (perhaps 5-7% in psychiatry), will take the
3 years of additional graduate specialty training (referred
to as aspirantura) leading to the degree of Candidate of
Medical Sciences (roughly equivalent to a Ph.D.). It is
from these ranks that professors and academic researchers
are chosen. The Doctorate of Medical Sciences, the highest

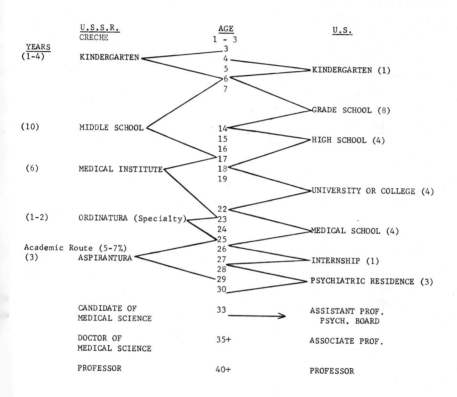

Figure 1. General and Medical Education

academic degree awarded in medicine, is given to a small
number of physicians, usually after many years of scholarly work and academic achievement.

Psychiatric training for a given trainee is largely
done in a single hospital, though there may be several
different assignments within the training to include some
experience in a neuropsychiatric dispensary. There are
some major differences in the approach to training from
that of American psychiatrists. Emphasis is upon learning
to recognize psychopathological signs and symptoms. Experience tends to emphasize diagnosis and psychopharmacologic
management of patients. Psychotherapeutic, or sociothera-
peutic modalities of treatment are not emphasized. Interpersonal dynamic formulations are minimized and psychiatric
problems are conceptualized primarily by altered manifest
behavior. An organic model of etiology for schizophrenic
illness is used. Psychosocial factors, particularly the
possible effect of a family upon a patient's illness are
minimized.

A sharp division is made in the Soviet Union between
psychiatric training and research. Psychiatric training
is totally clinical and is taught by practicing psychiatrists in the large mental hospitals. Research is carried
out by scientists who are not involved in teaching, and
whose full-time activities in research are in the psychiatric research institutes, independent of the medical institutes where students are trained. By contrast also, the
orientation in the Soviet Union is for each psychiatric
institute to concentrate on in-depth research in a single
area. The genetic and immunologic studies of schizophrenia
by the Psychiatric Research Institute, Academy of Medical
Sciences in Moscow are a good example.

PSYCHIATRIC PRACTICE

Psychiatry is a specialty of medicine in the Soviet
Union and is a wholly separate field from psychology.
Psychology itself is divided into two areas: neurophysiological research, and clinical psychological research.
The clinical area provides primarily for the study of brain
function in patients with neurological defects, but there
is no clinical testing or participation in treatment of
psychiatric patients by clinical psychologists. There is
also not a specialty of Social Work. Nursing is practiced

largely at a vocational level and the nurses on psychiatric
wards are not highly skilled mental health professionals.
The nurse is not encouraged nor trained to develop a therapeutic ward environment. She largely administers psychotropic drugs and maintains the patients' physical care.
They do, however, often take additional training and become
occupational therapists. The psychiatrist must carry out
many functions that are done by other mental health professionals in America (3).

Several differences occur in psychiatric practice,
due in large part to the fact that psychiatric services are
comprised in one system in the USSR. The Soviet health
care system provides geographically placed health dispensaries for the front line of medical care which is free
and readily accessible to patients. These general clinics
refer patients to specialized dispensaries. Neuropsychiatric dispensaries are provided for care of psychiatric
problems of an ambulatory nature in a population similar
to that served by an American community mental health
center. The neuropsychiatric dispensary accomplishes
continuity of care by the psychiatrist and nurse who provide all ambulatory and emergency psychiatric care to a
fixed population. The patient has a different physician
when hospitalized as an inpatient, though he may well return to the same psychiatrist at the dispensary. Alcoholism,
emergencies, child and adolescent problems, mental retardation, speech and neurological problems, such as epilepsy,
are treated there. They also function as day hospitals and
work therapy centers. Several dispensaries which are responsible for the population in a given geographic area
admit their patients to a central psychiatric hospital
designated for that area. Psychiatric hospitals tend to
be large facilities, containing several thousand patients
on multiple wards of 50 to 100 patients each. Psychiatric
hospitalizations are longer in the Soviet Union and may
be recommended more often than in the United States where
current emphasis is upon maintaining the patient in his
home environment as long as possible.

The single care system in the Soviet Union leads to
rapid and efficient early detection of mental illness, as
well as assured follow-up of the patient upon discharge
from the hospital back to the neuropsychiatric dispensary
in his area. It is thus quite unlike the American system
which has no central authority and no mechanism to insure

continuity of care or follow-up when a patient moves from
one level of care to another.   There is considerably less
emphasis upon the mental patient's legal rights in the
Soviet Union.   There is no constant legal review of patients
who are admitted, either voluntarily or involuntarily, to
ordinary mental hospitals, as occurs in the United States
by designation of an element of the judicial system to
defend the mental patient's civil rights.   Persons in the
Soviet Union who are accused of a crime, but are suspected
of having mental illness, are handled through a forensic
psychiatric system which functions quite separate from the
usual psychiatric hospitalization procedure (5).   They
would not be admitted to a regular mental hospital, but
would go directly to a forensic unit.

        Emergency services in the USSR are highly organized
into a single system.   Rapid identification and attention
to a psychiatric problem which occurs in home, factory or
public place is carried out by the emergency ambulance
service.   The emergency service provides a psychiatric
evaluation of any person identified as behaving irrationally
at home or at work.   Only the psychiatrist can make a determination of the need for a patient to be admitted to a
psychiatric hospital, and only he can sign papers for admission.   Signs of mental disturbance are sufficient for
hospitalization without requiring the presence of symptoms
which indicate possible danger of the patient to himself or
others.   Involuntary admission occurs when both the patient
and family refuse to accept the psychiatrist's decision to
admit the patient to the hospital, otherwise the admission
is deemed a voluntary one for the patient.

        Psychopharmacologic treatment is widely used for
psychiatric illness and the psychotropic drugs are used
with a high degree of skill.   The same psychotropic drugs
are used at similar doses as those in the US, with heavy
reliance on phenothiazines for schizophrenic patients and
lithium for manic-depressive psychosis.   Greater reliance
is placed upon intramuscular use of the phenothiazines,
especially during the early treatment phase of hospitalized
schizophrenic patients.

        Emphasis on the psychotherapeutic (individual and grou
approach to all patients, both hospitalized and ambulatory,
is minimal in the Soviet Union.   Families are not actively

involved in treatment or in discharge planning. The use of
family therapy is absent. There is, however, increasing
emphasis on rehabilitation, particularly in Leningrad, and
the use of collective psychotherapy which utilizes group
pressure to alter a patient's behavior. Electroshock is
used extremely conservatively; insulin coma is used to some
degree, but much less than in the past.

CONCEPTS OF MAJOR MENTAL ILLNESS

Both Russian and American psychiatrists generally
share the concept that major mental illness (schizophrenia,
and manic-depressive psychosis) likely has a dual etiology:
biological and environmental. However, the emphasis in
clinical treatment in the USSR is biological, whereas in
the United States it is largely on the environmental aspect.
In the USSR, the anamnesis reflects concern for genetic
factors by taking a careful genealogical history but with
little description or history of interpersonal relationships. Psychopathological signs in the USSR are much more
carefully defined descriptively and and great emphasis is
placed on determining the precise diagnosis. By contrast,
in the United States, less time is devoted to details of
diagnosis and more discussion is given to the therapeutic
intervention.

The group at the Institute of Psychiatry in Moscow
have developed a classification of schizophrenia which
determines the subtypes by the clinical course of the disease, as well as by the presenting psychopathological
signs (6). The American classification (American Psychiatric Association Diagnostic Manual II) is based primarily
on presenting psychopathological signs with less attention
to the clinical course which the illness has followed.

This concept of classification has evolved in the
Soviet Union as a modification of Kraepelinian classification of schizophrenia. In the 1930's, Sukhareva (8) described three forms of schizophrenia which she observed in
children, based on the clinical course: continuous,
periodic or recurrent, and a mixed form with characteristics
of both. Melekhov (4) extended the observation to adults,
calling the middle form "shift-like" (meaning occurring in
attacks but without full remission). Snezhnevsky and his
group have studied and elaborated these three types:

continuous, shift-like and periodic forms. Three subtypes
can be found in both the continuous and shift-like forms,
determined by the rapidity of the downhill course and the
presence of characteristic symptoms (7). The continuous
form has a malignant type characterized by simple and hebephrenic symptoms, a moderate type characterized by predominantly paranoid symptoms, and a sluggish (slow) type in
which symptoms are pseudoneurotic, or what might be called
latent or borderline symptoms in other classifications.
The shift-like form contains a severe subform, characterized
by catatonic symptoms, a moderate paranoid subform, and a
mild pseudoneurotic subform. The periodic form has acute
schizoaffective symptoms and is followed by full remission
and has a good prognosis. The advantage of this system,
as developed by Professor Snezhnevsky and his group, is
that this classification allows one to make a diagnosis
which will not change, which has prognostic values, and
which may be closer to basic etiologic aspects of the
disease. The concept of a genuine versus schizophreniform
illness or nuclear versus reactive form of schizophrenia
often has been proposed, which is thought to predict a
different course, outcome, and even etiology. The Soviet
classification may constitute independent observation in
the same direction, supporting the need for more careful
look at delineation of forms of schizophrenia by clinical
course and symptomatology.

In the Moscow School developed by Snezhnevsky, the
use of the word schizophrenia constitutes a broader "um-
brella" than in the United States, encompassing patients
who would be called borderline or latent schizophrenia
here. Also, schizophrenia is diagnosed more readily in
children and adolescents than in the US where we often
avoid using the term in younger patients and tolerate a
considerable degree of psychopathology in adolescents
under the rubric of adjustment reactions. This is not
true in the Soviet Union.

SUMMARY

Soviet psychiatrists specialize earlier in their medical careers than American psychiatrists. In the USSR most nonacademic psychiatrists begin to practice psychiatry after spending a year of training in a psychiatric hospital. Training concentrates on developing diagnostic acumen and developing skills in the use of psychopharmacologic and organic therapies. Psychotherapy, group and family therapy are not commonly used. Psychiatry is taught and practiced in geographically separate psychiatric hospitals. Psychiatrists have no other professional groups to utilize in psychological care of patients, except for nurses, who are trained primarily for physical aspects of care.

The single system of health care has supported development of emergency services and good integration of hospital and aftercare facilities. The neuropsychiatric dispensaries function as excellent community-based centers for care of ambulatory psychiatric problems.

A different subtyping of schizophrenia places emphasis upon clinical course, and broadens the use of the term, both at earlier ages and in latent and borderline patients. This concept deserves further study as a possible representation of etiologic differences.

Increasing interchange of American and Soviet psychiatrists, in both clinical and research areas, will be useful. An exchange will promote a more extensive evaluation of the similarities and differences in training, systems of psychiatric care, and concepts in the two countries. A cross-cultural appraisal of strengths and weaknesses in both systems should be advantageous to improved care of the psychiatric patient in both countries.

BIBLIOGRAPHY

BRONFENBRENNER, U.   Theory and research in Soviet character
    education.   Chap. VII in A. Simurenko (Ed.) Social
    Thought in the Soviet Union.   Chicago: Quadrangle
    Books, 1969.

HOLLAND, J.   "State" hospitals in the U.S.S.R.: A model of
    governmental psychiatric care.   In J. Zusman and E.
    Bertsch (Eds.) The Future Role of the State Hospital.
    Lexington, Mass.: Lexington Books, 1975.

HOLLAND, J., & SHAKHMATOVA, I.   Concept and classification
    of schizophrenia in the Soviet Union.   Schizophrenia
    Bulletin, in press, 1976.

MELEKHOV, D. E., SHUBINA, S. A., KOGAN, S. E., et al.
    Shizofreniya s istericheskimi proyavleniyami (Schizo-
    phrenia with hysterical manifestations).   In: Trudy
    Instituta imeni Gannushkina (Proceedings of the
    Gannushkin Institute), Vol. 1.   Moscow, 1936.   P. 91.

MOROZOV, G. V., & KALASHNIK, I. M. (Eds.).   Forensic
    Psychiatry.   White Plains, N.Y.: International Arts
    and Sciences Press, 1967.

NADZHAROV, R. A.   Formy techeniya, glavnye stadii razvitya
    shizofrenii i ee klinicheskie varianty (The clinical
    picture, main stages in the development of schizo-
    phrenia, and its clinical varieties).   In A. V.
    Snezhnevskii (Ed.), Shizofreniya (Schizophrenia).
    Moscow: Akademiya Meditsinskikh Nauk SSSR, 1972.

SNEZHNEVSKY, A. V.   Symptomatology, clinical forms and
    nosology of schizophrenia.   In J. D. Howells (Ed.),
    Modern Perspectives in World Psychiatry.   Edinburgh,
    London: Oliver and Boyd, 1968.

SUKHAREVA, G. E.   Klinika shizofrenii u detei i podrostkov
    (Clinical Aspects of Schizophrenia in Childhood and
    Adolescence).   Moscow, 1937.   P. 361.

PSYCHOTHERAPY IN THE USSR

Isidore Ziferstein

1819 North Curson Avenue
Los Angeles, California 90046

THE ROOTS OF RUSSIAN PSYCHOTHERAPY

Soviet writers on the history of medicine and psychiatry consider that a distinctive feature in the development of Russian and Soviet psychotherapy is its intimate interrelationship, from the very beginning, with medicine and physiology.

Authors like T. I. Yudin (1951), M. S. Lebedinskii (1971), N. V. Ivanov (1954), and others maintain that "in contrast to the main currents in foreign psychotherapy, Russian psychotherapy developed not in isolation from other fields of medicine and from physiology."

These writers trace the physiological and philosophically-materialist orientations of Russian psychotherapy to the profound influence of the philosophical writings of leading Russian thinkers of the nineteenth century like V. G. Belinskii, A. I. Gertsen, N. A. Dobrolyubov, D. I. Pisarev, and N. G. Chernyshevskii. Pavlov (1953) writes in his autobiography that he and his comrades were very much under the influence of these thinkers and were directed by these influences toward an interest in the natural sciences, very much the way Freud writes, in his autobiography, that "It was hearing Goethe's beautiful essay on Nature read aloud at a popular lecture by Professor Carl Brühl just before I left school that decided me to become a medical student." (Freud, 1959, p. 8).

The liberal Russian thinkers and philosophers of the
early and middle nineteenth century carried on a continuous
polemic against the prevailing idea of the duality of body
and soul. In a letter to V. P. Botkin, the elder brother
and mentor of the great Russian physician S. P. Botkin,
Belinskii wrote in 1847, "We must not separate the spiritual
nature of man from his physical nature, as though the former were something peculiar and independent from the latter."
(Lebedinskii, 1971, p. 76).

Yudin, Lebedinskii, et al state in their medico-histor-
ical writings that "the struggle of these remarkable Russian
philosophers-materialists for materialist principles which
merged with their democratic and revolutionary convictions,
influenced the formation of the theoretical views of Russian
physicians of the nineteenth century, as was noted later by
I. P. Pavlov." (Lebedinskii, 1971, p. 76).

These historiographers of Russian medicine, psychiatry,
and psychotherapy conclude that the relationship between
these disciplines was particularly intimate in Russia because the founders of Russian scientific clinical medicine
and surgery also laid the foundations for scientific psychotherapy in Russia. And that, indeed, the teachings of the
philosophers about the unity of body and soul led these
early Russian physicians to conclude that both somatic and
psychological illnesses should be healed by combinations of
somatic and psychological means.

Lebedinskii writes: "The most distinguished representatives of Russian medicine and physiology did extraordinarily
much for the development of psychotherapeutic ideas. The
tendency to take full account of the psychic aspect of any
illness was characteristic of the leading figures of Russian
medicine. The scientific understanding of the role of the
psyche in the causation, course, and treatment of diseases
was actively developed for almost two centuries. In Russia,
as nowhere else, the most prominent figures in general medicine directly developed psychotherapy and advocated its uses
In this connection, it is worth noting that in 1794, Skiadan
the professor of philosophy and medicine of Moscow University, refuting the pronouncements of many authorities of his
day, pointed to the cerebral cortex as 'the abode of the
soul.' Skiadan noted that passions of the spirit may produce
both a harmful and a beneficent effect on the organism, and

he cited case histories of patients with various somatic illnesses who were cured by psychic influences." (Lebedinskii,
1971, p. 75).

Lebedinskii also cites the outstanding clinicist M. Ya.
Mudrov, who wrote, at the turn of the nineteenth century,
that "There are also spiritual medicaments, which heal the
body," and emphasized the importance of "knowing the patient
in all his relationships, and learning all the causes which
operate on his body and soul." Lebedinskii lists, among the
early Russian clinicists where were interested in the psychological aspects of the treatment of somatic illnesses,
"the great surgeon N. I. Pirogov, a student of Mudrov,"
S. P. Botkin, G. A. Zakhar'in, F. I. Inozemtsev, and V. A.
Manassein. Lebedinskii concludes that "the founders of Russian clinical medicine strove to inculcate psychotherapeutic
principles into the entire range of medical therapeutic
work." (Lebedinskii, 1971, pp. 79-83).

THE THREE THEORETICAL PILLARS OF SOVIET PSYCHOTHERAPY

Soviet psychiatrists attribute the development of
present-day scientific Soviet psychotherapy to the pioneering work of two leading psychoneurologists: S. S. Korsakov
(1854-1900) and V. M. Bekhterev (1857-1927), whose life spans
coincided with much of the life span of Sigmund Freud.

Korsakov and Bekhterev based their concepts of the cause
and cure of mental illness on the work of the "father of Russian physiology," I. M. Sechenov, author of a monumental work
Reflexes of the Brain (1863) and the forerunner of Pavlov.

Influenced by Sechenov's researches, Korsakov regarded
psychic activity as a complex series of reflexes, and he
concluded that derangements of the normal reflex activity of
the central nervous system underlie all mental disorders.
Korsakov's (1887) classical study, "On a form of mental disease combined with degenerative polyneuritis" (Korsakov's
syndrome), was undertaken as part of his efforts to confirm
the theory that psychopathology could be shown to be related
to malfunctions and lesions of the central nervous system.

Bekhterev's work proceeded along similar lines, as
shown in his magnum opus, Foundations of Reflexology (1917).

In addition, Bekhterev particularly emphasized the role of social and environmental factors in the causation and treatment of mental disorders, as may be seen in a later publication, Collective Reflexology (1921).

Both Korsakov and Bekhterev demonstrated great awareness of the significance of the therapeutic community (the "collective" of patients) as a factor in the treatment of hospitalized mentally ill patients. Bekhterev emphasized the necessity for active intervention by the therapist in the real life situation of the patient, including environmental manipulation and work therapy.

1. The Pathophysiology of Mental Disorders. The first theoretical pillar of Russian and Soviet psychotherapy, then, was the doctrine that all mental disorders are caused by disturbances of the normal reflex activity of the central nervous system. Based on the pronouncements of Sechenov, and applied in clinical psychiatric reaserch by Korsakov, this theory was given an experimental foundation by the work of I. P. Pavlov and his pupils. Pavlov and his co-workers devoted many years of intensive work to the painstaking and detailed study of a relatively simple reflex in dogs, the secretion of saliva in response to the presentation of food, or in response to stimuli which had established "a temporary nervous connection" with the stimulus of the presentation of food. On the basis of these, and subsequent more complex and sophisticated experiments, Pavlov and his collaborators developed a complicated theoretical structure, which attempts to account physiologically for all of the psychological phenomena observed in animals and man. In his later years, Pavlov devoted himself to applying the theoretical principles of his system to specific clinical psychiatric illnesses in man.

According to Pavlovian theory, all psychic activity of animals and man is in fact the physiological activity of the cortex of the cerebral hemispheres and of the nearest underlying subcortical structures. The basic unit of the psychic activity is the neural reflex arc, involving three parts: (1) the receptors and afferent nerves, (2) the central nervous system, and (3) the efferent nerves and effectors--in the same way that the neural reflex arc is the basic unit of all functioning of the entire nervous system. Pavlov (1951) writes:

"This real activity of the hemispheres and of the neighboring subcortex, which ensures for the organism as a whole a normal adaptation in its complex relations with the external world, should rightly be considered and called the higher nervous activity, determining the external behavior of the animal (instead of the previously used term of 'psychical'), thus distinguishing this activity from that of the other parts of the brain and spinal cord, which mainly control the reciprocal relations and integration of various parts of the organism. This latter activity should be termed the lower nervous activity."

According to Pavlov, this "real activity" of the cerebral hemispheres and neighboring subcortex, which "ensures the normal adaptation of the organism to the external world," consists of the elaboration, mediation, and extinction of conditioned reflexes. The organism is born with a number of preformed reflexes, which Pavlov calls unconditioned. Chains or complexes of these unconditioned, inborn, reflexes form what are known as instincts. Pavlov at one time divided these instincts into two groups: the sex reflexes or instincts, which insure the preservation of the species; and the self-preservative instincts, which serve to safeguard the survival of the individual organism.*

The unconditioned reflexes serve to adapt the organism to those features of the environment which are constant. They constitute the primary adaptive equipment of the organism. The adaptation of the organism to the constantly changing aspects of the environment is accomplished by the superimposition of conditioned reflexes upon the unconditioned

---

*Note the similarity to Freud's early classification of instincts. Also analogous to Freud's formulations is Pavlov's statement that "the subcortex is the source of energy for all of the higher nervous activity, while the cortex plays the role of a regulator in relation to this blind force, exquisitely controlling and restraining it. ...In the subcortical centers are preserved traces of unusually powerful stimulations of the past, and these traces make themselves known, as soon as there is a weakening of the inhibiting effect of the cerebral cortex on the subcortical centers" (Fiziologiya i patologiya vysshei nervnoi deyatel'nosti [Leningrad and Moscow: Gosmedizdat, 1930], pp. 32-33). This is very much like Freud's conception of the relationship between the ego and the id.

reflexes. Pavlov (1951) defines the conditioned reflex as "a temporary nervous connection between the innumerable agents of the environment and specific activities of the organism." This means that the organism now reacts not only to the original stimuli that were effective at birth (the unconditioned stimuli), but also to the myriad environmental stimuli which have established temporary connections with the unconditioned stimuli. In this way, these conditioned stimuli act as signals, representing the original unconditioned stimuli; and the capacity of the organism to interact with the environment is vastly enriched and refined as these temporary connections are constantly changed and corrected in response to changes in the environment.

The degree of successful adaptation will depend on the exquisiteness with which the making and unmaking of these "temporary connections"--the conditioned reflexes--is attuned to the environment; that is, on the accuracy and speed with which the conditioned reflexes can change in response to minute changes in stimuli coming from the environment.

Mental illness is basically a breakdown in the responsiveness of the reflex activity to changes in external reality. Breakdowns may occur in various areas of conditioned reflex activity, giving rise to a variety of symptom complexes.

Pavlov devoted the last years of his professional life to efforts to establish correlations between the generally accepted nosological psychiatric entities and specific types of breakdown of the physiology of the higher nervous activity. He did this partly by analogy with some of his experimentally produced neuroses in dogs (Pavlov, 1941), but mostly by direct study of human patients at the Balinskii Psychiatric Hospital in Leningrad (Pavlov, 1954-1957).

Thus, on the basis of studies of patients at the Balinskii Hospital suffering from hysteria, Pavlov and his coworkers formulated a series of conclusions relating to predisposing factors, pathogenesis, and therapy of this condition. They concluded that the individual who is predisposed to develop hysteria has a relatively weak cerebral cortex, i.e., the cells of the cortex are easily fatigued and therefore become subject to a protective inhibition of their activity. In this situation, the subcortical centers are relatively free from cortical control, and the patient may be

subject to violent affective discharges and primitive motor
reactions, which take the form of hysterical attacks or fits.
The high inhibitability of the cortex creates a favorable
soil for the emergence of a deep state of hypnosis and pro-
tracted torpor. On the other hand, the highly active subcortex may establish, by induction, isolated points of excitation in the cortex. Because of the state of inhibition
in the rest of the cortex, these isolated points of excitation are relatively free from cortical control. This explains the increased suggestibility and autosuggestibility
of patients suffering from hysteria. The mechanism here is
similar to the one that Pavlov postulated for hypnotic and
posthypnotic suggestion, where most of the cortex is in a
state of hypnotic inhibition and the hypnotist is able to
have a strong, direct influence on isolated cortical points
of excitation.

Another characteristic of persons prone to hysteria is
a relative weakness of the second signaling system. Pavlov
referred to two systems of signals which were effective in
producing conditioned reflexes. The first signal system consists of the direct sensations of objects in the environment, which, as Pavlov wrote, "are for us [and for animals]
the primary signals of reality, the concrete signals." The
second signal system is constituted by "speech, chiefly the
kinesthetic stimulations flowing into the cortex from the
speech organs, the signals of signals. They represent in
themselves abstractions of reality and permit of generaliza-
tions, which indeed make up our added special human mental-
ity, creating first a general human empiricism, finally
science--the instruments of the higher orientation of the
human in the environment and toward himself." (Pavlov, 1941,
p. 93). The relative weakness of the second signaling system
in the hysteric may cause it to sink into an inhibited state.
As a result, the signals of the first system, with their
imagery and concreteness, come into play with full force,
producing vivid fantasies which distort the perception
of reality, with fantasy and daydreaming, leading at times
to twilight states.

The question of the triggering mechanisms that will
cause a hysteria-prone person to decompensate and develop
an overt hysteria was answered in part by studying the factors which produced neuroses in dogs in the laboratory.
Pavlov and his co-workers, M. K. Petrova and V. V. Rikman,

found that previously healthy dogs could be made neurotic by
a variety of noxious influences, either somatic or psychogenic. The somatic influences included experimentally induced interferences with glandular functions, as well as
artificially induced infections and intoxications.

Petrova and Rikman discovered that a variety of noxious
psychogenic influences could precipitate neuroses in dogs.
These included general traumatic experiences like: subjecting the experimental animal to several unusual and powerful
stimuli simultaneously, e.g., an overwhelmingly loud noise,
a bizarre and threatening visual image, being swung violently
on a special platform, etc. A more specific psychogenic agent
was the introduction of inner conflict, by requiring the experimental animal to respond to painful electrical shocks not
by the normal unconditioned defensive reflex but by a conditioned reflex of licking the food platter. In this case, the
dog suffered a neurotic breakdown when the painfulness of
the shocks exceeded a certain strength.

Most significant was the production of experimental
neuroses by requiring of the dog excessively delicate dis-
criminations, which were beyond its capacity. For example,
the dog was required to respond one way when it was shown a
circle, and in exactly the opposite way when it was shown
an ellipse. In successive experiments, the ellipse was gradually made to look more and more like a circle. At first,
the experimental animal had no difficulty making the discrimination, and continued to respond as it had been conditioned. However, at a certain point, the dog was no longer
able to discriminate between the two stimuli, and the resulting conflict produced a neurotic breakdown, which in
many ways resembled human hysteria.

By subjecting dogs with varying predispositions to the
experimental conditions described above, Pavlov and his co-
workers produced various types of breakdowns which resembled
various human neuroses and psychoses. Pavlov considered
these experimentally produced illnesses in dogs to be rough
and simplified models of mental illness in humans (Ivanov-
Smolenskii, 1949).

It is worth noting that Pavlov was well aware of the
connection between this work and Freud's psychoanalytic investigations. In 1935, Pavlov was visited in his laboratory
by Dr. Ralph W. Gerard, an American researcher.

They were discussing his work on conditioning and especially the production of experimental "neuroses" in dogs
by presenting them with a task of discrimination which was
too difficult. To Dr. Gerard's surprise, Pavlov said with a
twinkle, "Do you know that I was led to try these experiments by reading some of Freud's work?" He then proceeded
to speak of his indebtedness to Freud for stimulating his
thoughts and his experiments into this productive channel,
and added that he anticipated that deeper understanding of
behavior would come from a fusion of the concepts of the
conditional reflex and of psychoanalysis (Kubie, 1964,
pp. 202-203).

Another nosological entity, obsessive-compulsive neurosis, was explained by analogy to a particular type of experimental neurosis produced in dogs. Pavlov (1935) writes:

"With our pathogenic techniques, by which we make the
entire cortex pathological, it is also possible to produce
illness in a completely isolated region of the cortex. This
is an extraordinarily important and highly impressive fact.
Consider a dog with a series of different acoustic conditioned stimuli: beats of a metronome, a noise, a tone, a
crackling sound, a gurgling sound, etc. It is not difficult
to bring about a state in which only one of all these stimuli will be pathogenic, and will evoke a sharp deviation
from the normal."

This "sick point" may then be characterized by a state
of "pathological inertness," which means that it is no
longer possible by the usual methods to extinguish the conditioned reflexes related to stimulation of this area of
the cortex, and such conditioned reflexes may then persist
for years. Pavlov drew an analogy between the characteristics of such a "sick point" in his experimental animals
(with its isolation from the rest of the cortex and excessive stability of its pathological reactions) and obsessive
phenomena in humans, which are often isolated "pathological
points" in an otherwise relatively unchanged mental activity.
In his work with human patients, Pavlov found that obsessive-
compulsive individuals demonstrate, in addition, a marked
predominance of the second signal system (the verbal, intellectual aspects of the personality) over the first signal
system (the sensuous, concrete, emotional aspects).

Pavlov and his co-workers carried out similar investigations of manic-depressive psychosis, paranoia, neurasthenia,
psychasthenia, catatonic schizophrenia, hebephrenic schizophrenia, delirium, etc. These investigations are being continued, and have had a significant impact on the treatment
of mental illness in the Soviet Union. For example, the Soviet psychotherapist invariably employs, in addition to psychotherapy, various drugs, the use of which is determined by
whether there is thought to be a predominance of excitation
or inhibition; whether the nervous system is in need of protective inhibition; whether roborant or tonicizing substances are indicated, etc. The use of prolonged sleep therapy
is explained, on the basis of Pavlov's teachings, as providing protective inhibition to nerve cells that have been
traumatized by excessive stimulation (Andreev, 1960). In my
observations of psychotherapy, I found that Soviet psychotherapists avoided direct confrontation or interpretations
of the patient's latent negative feelings or attitudes. Instead, the therapist would find a way to give the patient a
countervailing positive suggestion. It was explained to me
that, in accordance with Pavlov's findings, making a patient
conscious of fears and other negative feelings has an anti-
therapeutic effect, since it reinforces the already existing
unhealthy pattern that has been formed in the patient's
higher nervous activity; and that such negative reinforcement is particularly strong when it comes from the authori-
tative person of the therapist. (Ziferstein, 1965).

2. Dialectical and Historical Materialism. Professor
Evgenii Popov (1961, p. 422), a member of the Academy of
Medical Sciences of the USSR, summed up the significance of
Pavlov's work for psychiatry as follows:

"Thus Pavlov's teaching is important for psychiatry
primarily in that it has opened before us the possibility
of physiological, strictly objective investigation of the
most complex cerebral phenomena which were formerly considered accessible to analysis only from the subjective
psychological point of view. At the same time his discov-
eries prove the correctness and fruitfulness of the materialist approach to the study of the psychic and confirm
that 'the psychical, the mind, etc., is the highest product
of matter (i.e., the physical); it is a function of that
particularly complex fragment of matter called the human
brain.' (V. I. Lenin, Materialism and Empirio-Criticism,
Foreign Languages Publishing House, Moscow, 1952, p. 233)."

This brings us to a consideration of the second theoretical pillar of Soviet psychiatry, the philosophical orientation of dialectical materialism. The Soviet psychiatrist
is very much concerned with philosophical questions. He appears to be more knowledgeable in this area than the American
psychiatrist, and he maintains that a "correct" philosophical
orientation is crucial; that an "incorrect" philosophical
foundation must lead to distortions in psychiatric theory and
practice. He attributes much of what he considers erroneous
in Western psychiatric theory and practice to false "idealist" philosophical underpinnings, or to lack of philosophical
clarity.

The Soviet psychiatrists with whom I worked pointed
out that the Russian intellectual tradition is deeply
grounded in materialist philosophy; that the leading Russian intellectuals, writers, scientists, philosophers, and
progressive political thinkers had for many generations
engaged in an uncompromising struggle for the philosophy of
materialism against the obscurantism of the tsarist regime
and its philosophically idealist state religion. And to
this day diamat (dialectical materialism) is an important
subject of study in all graduate schools in the country,
including schools of medicine.

The Soviet psychiatrist is, as he believes all scientists should be, philosophically a materialist. He asserts
that all mental phenomena are manifestations of the activity
of highly organized matter. He "struggles against" the
philosophic idealists, for whom mental processes are primary; who assert that we cannot be certain of the existence
of the material world and can know with certainty only our
perceptions of it and our ideas about it. The Soviet psychiatrist believes in the reality and primacy of matter.
He states that man's consciousness is a reflection of the
real, material world, and that this world would continue to
exist even if there were no one to perceive it or be conscious of it.

For example, V. N. Myasishchev (1958, pp. 7-8) writes:
"Without a scientific, materialist psychology, it is impossible to solve the problem of psychogenesis and psychotherapy. Modern Soviet psychology is developing on the foundation of the general theory of dialectical and historical
materialism and on the foundation of the teachings of I. P.
Pavlov. It takes as its point of departure the socio-

historical and natural historical understanding of man. ...
Man is not only an object, but a subject, whose consciousness reflects reality and at the same time transforms it."

Soviet psychiatrists attach great value to Pavlovian
conditioned reflex theory precisely because they consider
it the most fruitful approach to the study of man's psyche
as a complex manifestation of the activity of highly organized matter--the brain.

In emphasizing the importance of the "socio-historical
understanding of man," Soviet psychiatrists often accuse
Western psychiatrists, especially psychoanalysts, of being
one-sidedly preoccupied with the intrapsychic conflicts of
the patient, to the exclusion of social and neurophysiological factors. The Soviet psychiatrist stresses that the
social structure in which the individual is born and reared
is crucial in determining the way in which his neurophysiological functioning develops. For this reason, environmental
manipulation plays an important role in the Soviet psychiatrist's psychotherapeutic armamentarium.

3. Intrapsychic Conflicts and Dynamic Psychotherapy. In
addition to Pavlovian neurophysiology and Marxian dialectical
materialism, Soviet psychotherapy has a third basic theoretical aspect, the study of the intrapsychic conflicts and of
the personality of the patient as crucial factors in his illness. This theoretical interest is, of course, closely related to the practice of what we would call dynamic (or uncovering) psychotherapy.

Western behavioral scientists are generally under the
impression that dynamic psychotherapy is not practiced in
the Soviet Union. Many even have the impression that dynamic psychotherapy is proscribed there. These beliefs are
probably overdetermined. A major reason is the lack of communication between Western and Soviet behavioral scientists.

A second reason for Western belief that dynamic psychotherapy is not practiced or even tolerated in the Soviet
Union is the well-known opposition, even hostility, of Soviet psychiatry to psychoanalysis as a theory of human personality and as a healing art.

A third reason is the fact that until recently very
little could be found in the Russian neuropsychiatric journa

about dynamic psychotherapy. Joseph Wortis' comprehensive
study Soviet Psychiatry, which was published in 1950, and
Bruno Lustig's excellent surveys of Soviet psychiatry, published in 1955 and 1957, leave the reader with the distinct
impression that Russian psychiatrists employ somatic treatments almost exclusively, and that what little psychotherapy is practiced consists of hypnosis, suggestion, and similar techniques.

In the course of five research-sojourns in the Soviet
Union (the first in 1959 and the most recent in the fall of
1971), I learned that dynamic, uncovering psychotherapy is
a living and growing psychotherapeutic modality there. I
met psychotherapists who have practiced and taught this type
of psychotherapy for many years. Most of them were familiar
with Western writings on the subject.

That the interest in dynamic psychotherapy is growing
is attested to by the appearance in recent years of such
books as V. N. Myasishchev's Personality and the Neuroses
(1960), a collection of articles that had been published
between 1935 and 1960; Problems of Psychotherapy of Functional Disorders in the Sexual Sphere in Medical Practice,
by Professor N. V. Ivanov, of Gorky (1961); contributions
on "Psychotherapy Today" by A. D. Zurabashvili, of Tbilisi,
and others (1963); Problems of Psychotherapy, edited by
M. S. Lebedinskii, of Moscow (1958); The Neuroses and Their
Treatment by A. M. Svyadoshch, of Karaganda, Kazakhstan
(1971); The Word as a Physiological and Therapeutic Factor,
by K. I. Platonov, of Kharkov (1959); Essays on Psychotherapy, by M. S. Lebedinskii (1971); The Problem of the Unconscious, by F. V. Bassin (1968); Collective Psychotherapy,
by S. S. Libich (1974); Psychotherapy, by I. E. Vol'pert
(1972); Psychotherapy in Nervous and Mental Diseases, by
B. D. Karvasarskii et al (1973); Handbook of Psychotherapy,
by V. E. Rozhnov (1974); and others.

The fact that the authors of these works include some
of the best known and most highly regarded psychiatrists in
the Soviet Union, who have headed institutes in such widely
scattered places as Leningrad, Moscow, Gorky, Tbilisi (Georgia), Kharkov (Ukraine), and Karaganda (Kazakhstan), indicates that dynamic psychotherapy is not a localized, limited
phenomenon in the Soviet Union.

In this connection, I have noted over my years of observation of the psychiatric scene in the Soviet Union, that
there has been a gradual moderation of the attacks on psychoanalysis; and that recent works on psychotherapy have begun
to express an interest in unconscious mental processes, and
to note some positive contributions made by Freud and his
followers.

For example, at the All-Union Conference on Philosophical Problems of Higher Nervous Activity and Psychology,
held in Moscow in May, 1962, F. V. Bassin, while critical
of psychoanalysis, urged Soviet scientists to pay more attention to studies of the unconscious, in the following
words:

"The study of the unconscious has for a long time not
been given the attention which corresponds to the important
role played by these peculiar manifestations of mental activity. This underestimation of the theory of unconscious
psychic processes appears to have been an exaggerated, and
therefore inadequate, reaction to the pseudoscientific character that was attached to the theory of "the Unconscious"
by idealistic philosophy and by Freudism. As a result of
this, the correct development of these important problems
was held back for many years. Only now are we beginning to
appreciate to damage caused to both theory and clinical
practice by this unwarranted aloofness of dialectico-
materialistically oriented investigators from the scientific
examination of an important category of psychic and nervous
processes." (Bassin, 1963, pp. 425-426).

And in his monograph on "the Unconscious," Bassin
writes: "However, there is no doubt that in certain respects
Freud succeeded in substantially deepening our understanding of 'the unconscious,' when compared to the work of Mun-
sterberg, Prince, Ribot, Hart, even Janet, and others. Firs
of all, we must keep in mind his principle of 'cure by making the unconscious conscious' (the principle of eliminatin
the pathogenic influences of dissociated, or in the specifi
language of Freudianism, 'repressed' elements of the psyche
by including them into the system of conscious experiences)
the importance of which was unequivocally emphasized by
I. P. Pavlov. Accepting this principle, we thereby acknowledge both the fact of the existence of such 'dissociating'

elements, and also the possibility that they have a pathogenic effect on conscious psychic activity." (Bassin, 1968,
pp. 92-93).

Similarly, in the second edition of his book, <u>Neuroses
and Their Treatment</u>, Svyadoshch writes: "A positive aspect
of the writings of Freud is the fact that they called the
attention of scientists to the question of the influence of
the drives on psychic processes, and also to the question
of the unconscious; they demonstrated a number of concrete
manifestations of 'the unconscious,' such as slips of the
pen, slips of the tongue, and individual neurotic symptoms;
they pointed out the role of conflicts between 'duty and
desire' in the causation of neuroses; noted the phenomena of
sublimation of sexual energy, and of the repression of experiences (which lie at the foundation of, e.g., hysterical
amnesias); they put forth the principle of analytic therapy,
i.e., of treatment by bringing to light experiences of which
the patient had been unaware." (Svyadoshch, 1971, pp. 29-30).

THE CURRENT STATUS OF DYNAMIC PSYCHOTHERAPY

The interest in dynamic psychotherapy is not just a
recent development. As early as 1937, V. N. Myasishchev and
E. K. Yakovleva published a paper in a leading psychoneurological journal about the psychogenesis of visceral disorders, in which they included a great many case histories,
dating back over a period of many years, illustrating their
technique of "pathogenetic psychotherapy." (Myasishchev and
Yakovleva, 1937).

"Pathogenetic psychotherapy" was developed and taught
at the Bekhterev Psychoneurological Research Institute in
Leningrad by Vladimir Nikolaevich Myasishchev, a pupil of
Bekhterev. In the later years of the Stalin regime, with
the increase in repression, rigidity, and dogmatism,
Myasishchev and the Bekhterev Institute were subjected to
severe criticism, and even the threat of a purge. Fortunately
psychiatry was spared until the famous "joint session of the
two academies" (the Academy of Sciences of the USSR and the
Academy of Medical Sciences of the USSR) of June-July, 1950,
at which Soviet medicine and psychiatry were severely criticized for not applying the teaching of Pavlov rigidly
enough to their disciplines.

In a recent book Professor Myasishchev alludes to this period as follows: "Branded as anti-Pavlovian fabrications were any criticisms of dogmatism or any proposals that all elements of the organism and the various levels of the nervous system be taken into consideration in studying the regulation of the activities of the organism, without one-sided biologizing and without underestimation of social conditions. The ruling orientation in the 1950's not only did not further the development of physiology and pathophysiology of the nervous system, but it alienated and pushed aside realistically thinking theoreticians and clinicians from the ideas of nervism, and inflicted substantial damage to the development of a unified theory of medicine." (Myasishchev, 1966, p. 3).

Since Stalin died in 1953, and the process of "de-Stalinization" began almost immediately after Stalin's death, the onslaught on psychiatry was of relatively brief duration. Fairly soon voices began to be heard calling for a liberalization of attitudes. For example, Professor F. V. Bassin stated at a conference that scientific work had been adversely affected "by the general conditions created by the cult of Stalin's personality. This bred dogmatism in the social and natural sciences, an uncritical attitude toward scientific authorities, and the resort to meaningless quotations as a substitute for independent research. Instead of solving scientific problems in an atmosphere of free discussion among competent specialists, the declaration of theoretical postulates became more or less the rule." (Bassin, 1962).

Professor Bassin deplored the neglect of psychology and the overemphasis on biology. He criticized the neglect of other approaches, such as cybernetics, information theory and psychopharmacology, and stated: "The theory of higher nervous activity should not be considered as the only possible method for the study of the functions of the higher regions of the nervous system. Other approaches to the problem must also be used. ...Both method and theory should be developed not only through a variety of disciplines, but also on the basis of diversified positions and from the point of view of diverse trends." (Bassin, 1962).

In a recent article, three leading Soviet theoreticians declare that "to 'reduce' the manifestations of consciousness to their physiological foundations, whether we are dealing with psychopathology or psychology, is in principle unacceptable. The concept that physiological factors are general but not specific determinants of consciousness is made evident, for example, by all the data of contemporary psychopharmacology."

And they conclude: "For all these reasons, it is out of the question to attribute an exhaustive explanatory role to the physiological factors in elucidating all the aspects of consciousness." (Sarkissov et al, 1965, pp. 69-70).

Along with this liberalization of thought has come a greater understanding and tolerance for Western psychiatric works and a marked diminution in dogmatic criticism of them. For example, Meditsinskii rabotnik of May 25, 1962, reported that a high-level committee of psychiatrists "noted that name-calling and labeling in the past had unfortunately discouraged theoretical discussion, and that this must now be avoided at all costs. ... One of the members, Dr. B. I. Smulevich, held that the attitude toward foreign scientists was incorrect. They were being portrayed either as reactionaries or as vulgarizers of science. They are, however, often honest scientists who are seeking correct answers. Since it would be difficult for them to suddenly think along materialist lines, a friendly, tactful attitude should be taken toward them, and their work should be analyzed and criticized with conscientious accuracy."

An indication that this new spirit still prevails is a recent review in the S. S. Korsakov Journal of Neuropathology and Psychiatry of the book by Redlich and Freedman, The Theory and Practice of Psychiatry.

The reviewer writes: "The problems of the incidence, forms, clinical study, and treatment of drug addiction and alcoholism are given an interesting and, in connection with specific practical requirements, a more detailed exposition than in Soviet textbooks.

"Although the approach of the authors to 'the theory and practice of psychiatry,' to the clinical study of psychic illnesses, their pathogenesis and treatment, is in many ways different from the positions of Soviet psychiatry, we believe that Soviet readers will with interest acquaint themselves with this serious and informative work. This book gives an objective and full presentation of the currents and

views which prevail in contemporary American psychiatry, and
is an example of an interpretation of psychic disorders which
differs from ours, but which is integrated and consistent.
The authors obviously have mastery over the entire many-sided
experience of the scientific study of the psychoses, although
this experience is subjected to a one-sided interpretation."
(Shternberg, 1967).

This new, flexible orientation of Soviet theory has
vindicated the various schools of dynamic psychotherapy in
the Soviet Union, and has given impetus to their continuing
development.

The basic approach of one of these schools, "pathogenetic
psychotherapy" (whose work I observed), is summed up by
Professor Ekaterina K. Yakovleva of the Bekhterev Institute,
in her monograph on obsessive-compulsive neuroses, as follows: "The pathophysiological mechanism of psychasthenia and
obsessive-compulsive states is elucidated by the works of
I. P. Pavlov and his school. However, the clinical investigation of these states, as of other neuropsychiatric illnesses, requires a knowledge not only of their pathophysiological basis, but also of the specific characteristics of
the psyche. Only by taking these into account can we understand the pathogenesis of the illness and work out a rational
system of treatment.

"The basic method of treating these illnesses is psychotherapy, combined with somatotherapy. Experience shows that
the most effective method of psychotherapy is deep or rational psychotherapy, a system which, in contradistinction
to other authors (Dubois, Freud, and others), stems from an
investigation of the real life history of the patient and
his experiences, and has the aim of restructuring the interpersonal relations and helping the individual toward a constructive resolution of his life problems." [Emphasis added]
(Yakovleva, 1958, pp. 135, 137).

OBSERVING "PATHOGENETIC" PSYCHOTHERAPY

During 1963-64, I spent thirteen months at the Bekhterev Psychoneurological Research Institute in Leningrad,
making direct observations of dynamic ("pathogenetic") psychotherapy as it was practiced there. By sitting daily in
the treatment rooms with patient and therapist, I had the

opportunity to follow the treatment of twelve different patients by five different psychiatrists.

Before going to the Soviet Union in 1963, I had spent two years making direct observations of psychoanalysis and psychoanalytic psychotherapy at the Institute for Psychiatric and Psychosomatic Research, Mount Sinai Hospital, Los Angeles.* A comparison of the two sets of observations revealed certain specific characteristics of Soviet dynamic psychotherapy, which will be discussed below. However, it would be instructive to begin with a clinical example of my Soviet observations, which I consider typical.

CLINICAL OBSERVATIONS

The patient was a woman of thirty-four, who was referred to the Bekhterev Institute from another city. (It should be noted that the Bekhterev Institute draws a fairly large percentage of its patients from other cities, and other republics of the USSR. The patients are hospitalized during their treatment at the Bekhterev Institute, and on discharge are referred for follow-up to the original referring agency.)

The patient's treatment was observed continuously during the entire period of her hospitalization of two and a half months. Her chief complaint was attacks of weakness, dizziness, "feeling bad," "legs feeling like cotton," which had begun three years previously and as a result of which she became increasingly afraid to go anywhere alone. The therapist was an older woman with many years of psychotherapeutic experience.

The sixth session of the treatment was a crucial one. In the course of this session, it became apparent to the observer that the therapist had carefully thought through a specific strategy, and was consistently pointing in that direction. The therapist's task was enormously complicated by the patient's talkativeness and circumstantiality, which served the patient as a formidable means of opposing the therapeutic goal set by the psychotherapist. For this reason,

---

*These observations were carried out as a part of a research project " A Study of the Psychotherapeutic Process," funded by the Ford Foundation, with Franz Alexander as Principal Investigator.

the session lasted for one and three-quarter hours. However, despite the resistance of the patient, the session produced definite therapeutic progress and an increase in insight, and proved to be a turning point in the patient's recovery.

The therapist begins the session by asking the patient whether, as a teacher, she's engaged in "vospitatel'naya rabota" (work dealing with the emotional problems and development of her pupils). This immediately establishes a positive atmosphere, in which the patient happily and proudly and very circumstantially tells of two instances of her successful work with two most difficult pupils.

The therapist then skillfully leads the patient to the conclusion that people's personalities can be changed not only in earlier years but also later in life. From this, the therapist guides the patient into a reexamination of personality traits in herself that she might consider it desirable to change. (This had already been the topic of a previous session.) The patient exclaims, "I forgot to mention a major fault--jealousy." She recalls, in this connection, an incident when a girl friend did not invite her to a football game but went instead with another girl. The patient refused to talk to her friend for an entire year after this incident.

At this point, the therapist gives a crucial genetic interpretation: she links the patient's present trait of jealousy with her jealousy of her younger brother, who was born when the patient was five years old, at which time she could not bear to give up her privileged position of only child. The therapist here refers to material that had already been earlier obtained, e.g., that the patient occasionally stepped on her brother's hands when he began to crawl. That this interpretation hits the mark is demonstrated by the patient's producing confirmatory associations; for example, she recalls that she would forcibly turn her grandmother's face toward herself when the latter tried to talk with other people, instead of devoting exclusive attention to the patient.

The therapist now ties this up with a major present-day life problem, which the patient considers to be a main source of her illness: her seemingly insoluble life-and-death struggle with her husband's parents. The therapist asserts that, while it is doubtless true that the in-laws are very difficult people, the patient's jealousy and wish to have her husband all to herself play a major role in her conflict with them, and especially in the fact that the patient reacts so excessively and with such severe neurotic symptoms to this conflict. The therapist suggests that it should be possible for the patient to learn to live in the same town even with such "bad people" as her in-laws, without getting sick over it.

At this point, the patient's resistance, which until now has been covert, manifesting itself as excessive talkativeness under the guise of the wish to be cooperative and tell all, assumes an overt, outspoken, conscious form. The patient's face assumes a hard, set expression. She looks down grimly, and refuses to look up at the therapist. She weeps, in a combination of pique, anger, and self-pity, as during most of the remainder of the session she makes vehement statements that under no circumstances could she consider reconciling herself in any way to "those people"; that she would sooner leave her husband and live alone than do that; that perhaps the best thing, after all, is for her and her husband and child to move to another city. She reiterates that her husband's relatives exercise an evil influence over him; that as a result of their promptings he even began on occasion to beat her and the child, apparently to show that he was boss. She continues to produce examples to show that her in-laws are simply impossible to reason with, and she reiterates several times that she has no intention of reconciling herself to them.

It was clear at the time, and the further course of the therapy confirmed this, that this session probed into a fundamental character trait which lay at the basis of the patient's neurosis. The attempt to demonstrate to the patient that her illness is determined primarily by her personality and not by external circumstances or other people, and that therefore getting away from these circumstances will not solve her problem, arouses the most extreme opposition. The patient refuses absolutely to consider any approach that would involve her learning to get along with her husband's parents.

Both for a Soviet and for an American psychotherapist this kind of resistance becomes a major obstacle, which

will not be overcome in one or two sessions. But there is a
difference in the approaches employed in coping with this
resistance.

How did the Soviet psychotherapist accomplish it in this
case? Recognizing that there has been a change in the climate
--that the patient now has a negative attitude toward the
therapist and the therapy--the therapist decides, as a first
move, to regain the patient's positive feelings. These moves
are initiated in this (the sixth) session, and are continued
in subsequent sessions. Seeing that the patient is in a very
upset state, the therapist looks lovingly at the patient,
pats her hand, and says with great compassion, "We have quite
exhausted you, poor dear!" The therapist then takes the patient's hands in both of hers, and in a characteristic gesture moves them toward herself, thus bringing the patient
closer to her and almost forcing the patient to look up at
her while saying, "Tomorrow we will have a detailed discussion of the way it is possible to have a good life with your
husband and child, and at the same time not get into these
terrible conflicts over the in-laws" (a promise of positive
help and guidance). The therapist concludes the session with
a supportive, reassuring statement, "Your husband loves you,
and you do love him," as she again pats the patient's hands
and looks lovingly into her eyes. However, the patient has
the last word. She is willing to grant that her husband
loves her, but is rather dubious about the latter half of
the therapist's statement, i.e., that she loves him: "Let
us suppose I do love my husband. I simply cannot put up with
people like his parents and sister."

The interplay between patient's resistance and therapist's efforts to overcome it continues for many sessions.
One example: In the following session, the therapist points
out to the patient that she is meeting with her as her first
patient in the morning. This is a kind of peace offering--
a gift to the patient's need for some mark of special recognition. But the patient's resistance is mounting. She counters by complaining of more severe vertigo. She tells a
dream:

"I saw a funeral procession. A woman was lying in a cof-
fin, with her hand up in the air, and electrodes connected
to it." Association: "The woman had died as the result of
an electroencephalogram." (The patient had had an EEG

just before Session VI, and she is saying, "This treatment
will kill me!") The therapist does not interpret, but responds
and counters with, "You're a socially aware and active person. You're involved in the rearing of the young, in whom we
attain immortality." (The therapist is saying, "No, the therapy will not kill you--it will help you attain immortality!") "Pedagogues are the most important people." (I found
that often therapists, while not verbally interpreting a
dream, responded to its latent content, as in this example.)

In general, one can classify the therapist's efforts
under three headings:

1. Efforts to maintain a positive therapeutic climate by
demonstrating to the patient great interest and concern, respect and appreciation for the patient's positive qualities.
For example, in Session XII, the patient complains that the
Director of her school is creating difficulties for her. He
has written to her to say that she may not stay away from
school for her treatment longer than a month unless she re-
ceives a special document from the therapist. The therapist
utilizes this opportunity to tell the patient that this is
proof that the Director values her highly and is therefore
simply trying to exert pressure to get her back as soon as
possible. Here again an interplay with the patient's resis-
tances takes place. The patient counters this move by saying
that one doctor told her she had a weak nervous system and
should not be engaged in so taxing an occupation as teaching,
that she should change to library work. The therapist expresses great horror at such a suggestion. She again vigor-
ously assures the patient that she is uniquely equipped to
be a teacher, and that it would be a great loss if the patient were to leave the profession of teaching.

2. Efforts to help the patient by direct advice and
guidance on how to handle her life problems in a more mature, realistic, healthy manner. These include, for example,
detailed discussions of how the patient reacts, and how she
should react, when her friends report to her the slurring
remarks her in-laws make about her.

3. Interpretations of patient's neurotic behavior and
symptoms, and confrontation with her opposition to psychotherapy. For example, when the therapist points out to the
patient that she is not cooperating in the treatment, the

patient protests that, on the contrary, she is, and always
has been, very cooperative. The patient cites, as an example,
that when she was in another hospital she readily submitted
to all the injections, although she is very much afraid of
being stuck with needles. The therapist then points out that
the patient is much less resistive to the physical pain of
somatic treatment than to the psychic pain of gaining insight. Of these three types of intervention, the first two
are the most prominent.

These efforts by the therapist proved effective. Gradually, the therapist was able to achieve her aim of restoring
a positive relationship and significantly reducing the patient's resistance. Eventually, after two and a half months
of treatment (thirty-eight therapeutic sessions), the patient
was discharged with significant symptomatic improvement, a
warmer attitude toward her husband, and a more reasonable
set toward the husband's parents. Follow-up reports, by letters from the patient, over the twelve years since discharge,
show that the patient is maintaining her improvement, and is
in fact making further progress.

(Of course, this was not all there was to the therapy.
The other psychotherapeutic aspects of the treatment, as
well as the extensive use of other adjunctive treatments,
will be described elsewhere.)

An American psychotherapist would have employed the same
three types of intervention: encouragement and support, re-
education, and interpretation. But the emphasis would have
been most heavily on the third--interpretation. In the case
of a psychoanalyst, the emphasis would be almost exclusively
on interpretation, with support and reeducation in very small
and indirectly expressed doses. The major effort in dealing
with the patient's resistance would be directed toward con-
fronting the patient with the fact that she is resisting,
demonstrating to her over and over again the variety of forms
that her resistance is taking, and eventually interpreting
the meaning and the sources of the resistance. For example,
in Session VII, when the therapist asks the patient whether
she had thought about what was discussed in Session VI, the
patient answers that she didn't give it any thought because
the therapist had told her that the discussion would be continued on the following day. Similarly, when the patient is
informed that the medication she has been receiving (Pheni-
gamma) is being discontinued because of her side-reactions

to it, she says, "Then that means I won't be getting any
treatment at all!"--thus completely negating psychotherapy
as a form of treatment. An American analytically oriented
psychotherapist would probably have confronted the patient
with these evidences of her resistance.

The dream about the woman killed by the EEG would
probably be used to demonstrate to the patient her mortal
fear of the therapy. Further associations might lead to uncovering a fear, perhaps, that her mother would kill her in
retaliation for her hostile feelings toward her brother. Ultimately, a transference-interpretation might be formulated
thus: "You want to be the therapist's only child," (with il-
lustrations from the patient's resentment of, and competition
with, the therapist's other patients) "just as you want to be
your parents' and in-laws' only child. You want to be the
central figure, standing between your husband and your parents, as well as between your husband and his parents." The
patient's major symptom of feeling giddy and unreal would
probably eventually be interpreted as a refusal to accept the
present reality, in which she is one among many, and a wish,
through her illness, to force the world to be different, to
force a return to the time before the brother was born, when
she was the only child.

CHARACTERISTICS OF SOVIET PSYCHOTHERAPY

The above example is typical of the material obtained
during more than a year of observation in 1963-64, and during subsequent studies carried out in 1970 and 1971. It il-
lustrates, in part, several outstanding characteristics of
the patient-therapist interaction in Soviet psychiatry and
psychotherapy.

1. Activity

The Soviet psychiatrist plays an active role in treatment, diametrically opposite to the non-directive, purely
interpretive role that is advocated by classical psychoanalysis. This activity is manifested in many ways. The psychiatrist may manipulate the patient's environment, his job,
his occupation, his place of work, or his place of residence,
if he considers these to be factors in the patient's illness.

The doctor will not only advise a change of job or residence. He will personally (not through a social worker) contact the appropriate authorities--the factory manager or the housing committee--to see that the prescribed changes are carried out.

This was illustrated in a case I observed in which the patient was a young factory worker. In the course of therapy, the psychiatrist and the patient arrived at the conclusion that a major factor in the patient's neurosis was the unchallenging, unrewarding nature of his work. The therapist felt that the patient had the capacity to become an engineer, and that this would help him develop into a competent, fulfilled, and healthy person. On discharging the patient, the doctor wrote a prescription, addressed to the factory director, which required that the patient be enrolled in an engineering institute, and that the factory pay his full salary during the entire period of his schooling. Such prescriptions are binding on the factory management.

In keeping with his position as the expert, as "the citizen who knows," the Soviet psychiatrist is "in charge" during the entire course of treatment. When conducting psychotherapy, the psychiatrist decides, after the first two or three exploratory sessions, what the patient's major problem areas are. He then discusses with the patient the goals of the treatment, and proceeds to direct and guide the content and form of each session, so as to deal systematically with each problem in turn.

Because of his collective upbringing and his "brother's keeper" orientation, the Soviet psychiatrist involves himself much more actively and with much more emotional cathexis in his patients than the psychoanalysts I have observed in this country.

The importance of active, emotionally cathected involvement by the psychiatrist has been enunciated as a major principle of Soviet psychotherapy by its leading theoreticians. G. A. Gilyarovskii (1959) writes that psychiatric treatment "requires not only a kind, loving attitude toward the patient. It also requires active intervention in his life and the lives of the people around him. ... The Soviet doctor is not an observer, but an active friend and servant of those who suffer."

Another leading Soviet psychiatrist, Professor V. N. Myasishchev (1960, p. 378), formerly director of research at the Bekhterev Institute, writes:

"The relationship of the patient to the doctor is most important and decisive. This relationship becomes an effective force only when it acquires a positive emotional character. The authority of the doctor, the trust, esteem, and love of the patients for him, are not acquired at once, but gradually, as the doctor, by his skillful approach to the patient, helps him to gain an understanding of his life story, of the complicated, confused, ununderstood and misunderstood circumstances of his past and present."

The Soviet psychiatrist believes that it is the doctor's responsibility to maintain a positive climate in the therapy --a climate in which the patient develops "trust, esteem, and love" for the doctor. If the climate is not positive, or if the patient develops negative feelings, this is considered to be the result of errors committed by the doctor. It is then the psychiatrist's responsibility to take active steps to gain or regain the patient's positive feelings.

The Soviet psychiatrist is therefore very active in giving the patient emotional support and building up the patient's self-esteem. The doctor does not hesitate to give the patient advice and guidance in his day-to-day problems. His efforts to reconstruct the unhealthy personality structure involve exploring its pathogenesis, but with the predominant emphasis on active reeducation, presenting to the patient those values and standards of behavior which are considered correct, realistic, and socially desirable.

Soviet psychiatrists are active themselves and they expect activity of their patients. The treatment received by patients at the Bekhterev Institute was active and vigorous, and was reminiscent of the "total push" program advocated in our country for the hospitalized mental patient. The patient's waking time was almost totally occupied with a variety of activities, and the mental illness was attacked on a variety of fronts simultaneously.

2. Work as a Healing Agent

A central part of this total-push approach is work therapy. On the grounds of the Bekhterev Institute are a number
of fully equipped factories in which several hundred patients
are employed. About half are inpatients. The rest are outpa-
tients living in the neighborhood of the institute. In these
factories, trained foremen as well as psychiatrists supervise
the patients in the production of such articles as furniture,
clothing, fountain pens, and hammocks. These articles are
sold under contract to retail stores, and the patients are
paid for their work.

The hours that the patient spends in the hospital factory, engaged in productive work, are considered a crucial
part of his treatment, and all patients who are physically
able are required to work.

Work therapy is considered by Soviet psychiatrists a
major tool in their therapeutic armamentarium, just as their
society looks upon work as a central element in the life of
every person, male or female; and their Marxist ideology
teaches that the evolution of man from ape was made possible
by the emergence of social labor, i.e., work that is carried
out cooperatively and that is socially useful.

Soviet psychiatrists emphasize that work therapy helps
to maintain the patient's contact with reality and to prevent emotional isolation and retreat from the real world;
that doing socially useful work, and getting paid for it,
helps restore and enhance the patient's self-esteem; and that
work under the protected conditions of the therapeutic work-
shop helps prepare the patient for a return to normal life
and work on the outside.

Some patients continue working in the protected hospital
workshops after discharge until such time as they are ready
to return to work under ordinary conditions. There are patients for whom the hospital offers an opportunity for re-
training in a new skill which suits them better and/or is
more highly paid.

I recall a patient who was assigned to work in the electronics shop. During the three months of his hospitalization,
he acquired considerable skill in assembling and repairing

electronic devices used in medical research. When he was
ready for discharge he asked and obtained permission to continue working in the electronics shop for several more months
to increase his skill. He finally became proficient enough
to obtain an interesting, highly skilled, and well-paid job
in industry. In a follow-up interview, I noted that for this
man there was no stigma attached to psychiatric hospitalization. He told me that he boasted to his neighbors and friends
about the high-status profession he had learned at the Bekhterev Institute.

3.   Somatic Therapies, Medication, Physiotherapy

As was indicated earlier, the Soviet psychiatrist has
been brought up in the tradition of a close, intimate interrelationship between psychology and neurophysiology and between psychiatry and medicine. He holds that an important
factor in all mental illness is a disturbance in the physiology of the central nervous system.

In keeping with this orientation, he draws no sharp distinction between psychotherapeutic, physiotherapeutic, and
pharmacotherapeutic approaches to the treatment of neurosis
and psychoses. From the moment of the patient's admission to
treatment, the Soviet psychiatrist becomes the patient's personal physician. As part of the first interview, the psychiatrist carries out a complete physical and neurological examination of the patient; and he diagnoses and treats whatever
somatic complaints or illnesses the patient may present,
calling in specialized consultants when indicated.

Throughout the course of treatment, the therapist employs, in addition to psychotherapy, a wide variety of psychotropic drugs. The Soviet psychotherapist does not look
upon drugs as foreign substances, but rather as a beneficent
agent which is intended to make up for whatever deficiencies
may exist in the central nervous system, by strengthening it,
tonicizing it, stimulating it, or producing a protective inhibition to protect it from overstimulation. Considerable
psychopharmacological research is now being carried out on
the use of synthetic substances which are analogues of fatty
acids found in normal brain tissue. The aim is to develop a
system of replacement therapy, i.e., supplementing substances
which should be normally present but are either absent or

deficient in case of illness, similar to the use of thyroid
extract in thyroid deficiency, and of insulin in diabetes.

The Soviet psychotherapist also uses, as adjunctive
treatment, various forms of hydrotherapy and physiotherapy,
including the ancient Chinese technique of acupuncture.

4. Availability and Accessibility

One manifestation of the Soviet psychiatrist's immersion
in the collective feeling, which is an important part of his
upbringing from early childhood, is the emphasis on informality and on availability of the doctor. The patients whose
treatment I observed were all hospitalized, and there were
no present appointments for psychotherapeutic sessions. Patients were seen at various times of the day, depending on
the schedule of the other treatments and activities. Sessions
were not limited to the fifty-minute psychoanalytic "hour,"
but varied quite informally in duration from one half hour
to two hours or longer. I was interested to find, moreover,
that this informality and easy availability of the therapist
applied not only to the hospitalized patients, but also to
former patients who occasionally wanted to see their former
psychiatrist.

This was brought to my attention dramatically one day
when I was observing a therapeutic session. The door suddenly
opened and, without knocking, a man poked his head into the
room. With no apology or preamble, he asked to see the doctor. I, the American observer, was the only one upset by this
invasion. The doctor and the patient remained quite unper-
turbed. The doctor quietly advised the intruder that she
would be able to see him in half an hour. I later learned
that the intruder was a former patient. The doctor did not
agree with my suggestion that the patient ought to have tele-
phoned in advance for an appointment. She felt it was an important part of the therapeutic relationship that the patient
should know that the doctor was available whenever needed.

The availability and accessibility of the psychiatrist
is enhanced by an important economic factor: the fact that
psychotherapy, like all psychiatric and medical care, has to
be made available to all in the population who need it, without cost, and without regard to the ability to pay.

5. Group Psychotherapy

Soviet writers on the history of psychotherapy point out that Korsakov and Bekhterev, the founders of modern Soviet scientific individual psychotherapy were also the founders of Soviet group psychotherapy, or "collective psychotherapy," as they call it, to distinguish it from the Western type of treatment in groups.

Collective psychotherapy developed simultaneously, and in conjunction with, scientific individual psychotherapy. It was strongly influenced by the contributions of the educator A. S. Makarenko, who did remarkable work in reeducating and rehabilitating the bands of homeless and parentless youth who roamed the country at the time. Makarenko, in his writings, emphasized the role in character formation, as well as in re-education and rehabilitation, of the collective, including the family, the peer group, the school, and the various social institutions.

Professor N. V. Ivanov (1966), Chief of the Department of Psychiatry at the Kirov Institute of Medicine in Gorky, draws the following distinction between Western group psychotherapy and Soviet collective psychotherapy:

"In place of the retrospective emphasis of group psychotherapy abroad, the Soviet psychotherapist is concerned with the active mobilization of the personality and its compensatory powers on the basis of the elaboration of new connections, the conditioning of nervous processes, and the objective of creating new, powerful dynamic structures, which, insofar as they are the more powerful, are capable, in accordance with the law of induction, of extinguishing and destroying the pathologically dynamic structures that have given rise to the illness."

Collective psychotherapy is practiced extensively both in outpatient and inpatient settings; always in conjunction with individual psychotherapy, and with the use of the other adjunctive therapeutic modalities enumerated earlier, especially collective work therapy. The combination of collective psychotherapy and collective work therapy has become one of the hallmarks of Soviet psychotherapy (Ziferstein, 1972).

In recent years there has also been an increasing use, in the Soviet Union, of psychodrama, conjoint marital therapy, and family therapy.

6. Use of the Collective

As is to be expected from one whose life is oriented toward the central role of the collective in the security system of the individual, in the satisfaction of his material and emotional needs, and in the furthering of his growth and development, the Soviet psychiatrist makes active and frequent use of the collective for therapeutic purposes. In the forefront of his awareness is a realization of his reciprocal interaction with his society: society employs his professional skills for the benefit of the overall social enterprise, and he uses society, its regulations and institutions, to assist him in his professional work with the individual patient.

The psychiatrist has a large number of collectives available for his therapeutic purposes. He often calls upon the patient's collective and other social institutions, in addition to the family, for help in obtaining an anamnesis. He depends on members of the collective to visit the patient, to maintain contact with him, to help keep up his spirits, and to prevent isolation and withdrawal from reality. When the patient is discharged, the doctor may write to the trade-union organization, giving suggestions and instructions about attitudes toward the patient which will help promote recovery.

In the case of patients hospitalized at the Bekhterev Institute, I was able to observe how, consciously and unconsciously, the staff used the collective as a therapeutic instrument. The patient's time was almost totally occupied with a variety of activities involving constant interaction with fellow patients and the staff. The emphasis was always on the collective as an inspirational, encouraging, supportive, pressuring, corrective, and reality-testing medium.

The clinical conference at which patients were presented to the entire staff, including Professor Myasishchev, was also used consciously and actively by the staff as a therapeutic aid. It was impressed on the patient that at the conference he was privileged to have the benefit of the

collective wisdom of the entire staff. The staff members in-
teracted with the patient in a way that was clearly intended
not only to clarify obscure points but also to have a direct
psychotherapeutic impact on the patient. And it usually did.
Weekly ward rounds by the entire staff were similarly used
to exert a collective therapeutic effect on the patients.

The Soviet psychiatrists' involvement in the use of the
collective and their inability to let anyone be a bystander
was illustrated dramatically in their relationship to me. I
had explained to the staff that my aim was to be a totally
nonparticipant observer. But both the patients and the psychiatrists seemed constitutionally unable to let anyone be
merely an observer. Verbally and nonverbally, patients and
therapists seemed constantly to be saying to me, "Don't just
sit there! Do something!"

Not infrequently during therapeutic sessions, either the
therapist or the patient would turn to me with, "Don't you
think so, Isidore Samuilovich?", "What do you think, Isidore
Samuilovich?", "How is this problem handled in your country?"
I finally came to realize that, willy-nilly, I had become a
participant member in a therapeutic collectif-à-trois, whose
aim, like that of other collectives, was to increase the
well-being of the individual and the collective.

BIBLIOGRAPHY

ANDREEV, B. V. (1960). Sleep therapy in the neuroses. Trans.
    by B. Haigh, Consultants Bureau, New York.

BASSIN, F. V. (1962). In: Meditsinskii rabotnik, June 12,
    1962, as quoted in Wortis, J., A "thaw" in Soviet psy-
    chiatry?, Amer. J. Psychiat. 119(6):586.

BASSIN, F. V. (1963). Soznanie i "bessoznatel'noe" [Con-
    sciousness and "the unconscious"]. In: Filosofskie vo-
    prosy fiziologii vysshei nervnoi deyatel'nosti i psi-
    khologii [Philosophical problems of the physiology of
    the higher nervous activity and of psychology]. USSR
    Academy of Sciences Publishing House, Moscow.

BASSIN, F. V. (1968). Problema bessoznatel'nogo [The problem of the unconscious]. Meditsina Publishing House,
Moscow.

BEKHTEREV, V. M. (1917). Obshchie osnovy refleksologii cheloveka [General foundations of reflexology in man]. Petrograd.

BEKHTEREV, V. M. (1921). Kollektivnaya refleksologiya [Col-
lective reflexology]. Petrograd.

FREUD, S. (1959). An autobiographical study. In: The Standard Edition of the Complete Psychological Works of
Sigmund Freud, Vol. XX, Hogarth Press, London.

IVANOV, N. V. (1954). Vozniknovenie i razvitie otechestvennoi psikhoterapii [The origins and development of Russian psychotherapy]. Unpublished doctoral dissertation,
Moscow.

IVANOV, N. V. (1961). Voprosy psikhoterapii funktsional'nykh
rasstroistv polovoi sfery vo vrachebnoi praktike [Prob-
lems of psychotherapy of functional disorders in the
sexual sphere in medical practice]. R.S.F.S.R. Ministry
of Health, Moscow.

IVANOV-SMOLENSKII, A. G. (1949). Ocherki patofiziologii
vysshei nervnoi deyatel'nosti [Essays on the pathophysiology of the higher nervous activity]. Moscow.

KARVASARSKII, B. D., V. M. VOLOVIK, R. A. ZACHEPITSKII,
S. S. LIBICH, and V. K. MYAGER, eds. (1973). Psikhoterapiya pri nervnykh i psikhicheskikh zabolevani-
yakh [Psychotherapy in nervous and mental diseases].
Bekhterev Psychoneurological Research Institute, Leningrad.

KORSAKOV, S. S. (1887). On a form of mental disease combined
with degenerative polyneuritis. Vestnik klinicheskoi i
sudebnoi psikhiatrii i nevrologii, 4(2).

KUBIE, L. S. Pavlov, Freud, and Soviet psychiatry. Quoted in
Lebensohn, Z. M. (1964), Pavlovian conditioning and
American psychiatry. Symposium No. 9, March, 1964.
Group for the Advancement of Psychiatry, New York.

LEBEDINSKII, M. S., ed. (1958). Voprosy psikhoterapii [Problems of psychotherapy]. Medgiz, Moscow.

LEBEDINSKII, M. S. (1971). Ocherki psikhoterapii [Essays on psychotherapy], 2nd ed. Meditsina Publishing House, Moscow.

LIBICH, S. S. (1974). Kollektivnaya psikhoterapiya nevrozov [Collective psychotherapy of the neuroses]. Meditsina Publishing House, Leningrad.

LUSTIG, B.(1955). Die sowjetische Psychiatrie, Berichte des Osteuropa-Instituts an der Freien Universität Berlin. Vol. 17, Berlin.

LUSTIG, B. (1957). New research in Soviet psychiatry. Medical series of the reports of the Osteuropa Institute of the Berlin Free University, No. 14, Berlin. (English translation issued in mimeographed form by the University of California at Los Angeles.)

MYASISHCHEV, V. N. and E. K. YAKOVLEVA (1937). O psikhogennykh vistseral'nykh narusheniyakh [On psychogenic visceral disorders]. Sovetskaya psikhonevrologiya, 13(3): 17-28.

MYASISHCHEV, V. N. (1958). Nekotorye voprosy teorii psikhoterapii [Some problems of the theory of psychotherapy]. In: Voprosy psikhoterapii [Problems of psychotherapy], ed. by M. S. Lebedinskii.

MYASISHCHEV, V. N. (1960). Lichnost' i nevrozy [Personality and the neuroses]. Leningrad University Press, Leningrad.

MYASISHCHEV, V. N. (1966). O razlichnykh formakh svyazi psikhogennykh i somatogennykh narushenii kak aktual'noi probleme meditsiny [On the various types of relationship of psychogenic and somatogenic disorders as a current problem in medicine]. In: Nevrozy i somaticheskie rasstroistva [Neuroses and somatic disorders], ed. by V. N. Myasishchev, Valentina K. Myager, and A. Ya. Straumit, Bekhterev Psychoneurological Inst., Leningrad.

PAVLOV, I. P. (1935). Eksperimental'naya patologiya vysshei nervnoi deyatel'nosti [Experimental pathology of the higher nervous activity]. Biomedgiz, Leningrad.

PAVLOV, I. P. (1941). Lectures on Conditioned Reflexes. Vol. II: Conditioned Reflexes and Psychiatry, trans. and ed. by W. H. Gantt, International Publishers, New York.

PAVLOV, I. P. (1951). Fiziologiya vysshei nervnoi deyatel'-nosti [Physiology of the higher nervous activity]. (Paper read at the International Physiological Congress in Rome, September 2, 1932). In: Polnoe sobranie sochinenii [Complete works], Vol. 3, bk. 21, Moscow and Leningrad.

PAVLOV, I. P. (1904). Autobiography. Moscow. Quoted in E. A. Asratyan, I. P. Pavlov, His Life and Work, Moscow, 1953.

PAVLOV, I. P. (1954-1957). Klinicheskie sredy [Clinical Wednesdays], in 3 volumes. USSR Academy of Sciences, Moscow-Leningrad.

PLATONOV, K. I. (1959). The Word as a Physiological and Therapeutic Factor. Foreign Languages Publishing House, Moscow.

POPOV, E. A. (1961). Pavlov's physiological teaching and psychiatry. In: I. P. Pavlov. Psychopathology and Psychiatry. Foreign Languages Publishing House, Moscow. p. 422.

ROZHNOV, V. E., ed. (1974). Rukovodstvo po psikhoterapii [Handbook of Psychotherapy]. Meditsina Publishing House, Moscow.

SARKISSOV (SARKISOV), S. A., F. V. BASSINE (BASSIN), V. M. BANCHTCHIKOV (BANSHCHIKOV), H. EY, and Ch. BRISSET (1965). Problème du rôle des conceptions neurophysiologiques en psychopathologie [The problem of the role of neurophysiologic concepts in psychopathology]. Revue de médecine psychosomatique 7(1):65-81.

SECHENOV, I. M. (1863). Refleksy golovnogo mozga [Reflexes of the brain]. Meditsinskii vestnik, nos. 47-48.

SHTERNBERG, E. Ya. (1967). Review of Redlich, F. C. and
    D. K. Freedman: The theory and practice of psychiatry.
    Zhurnal nevropatologii i psikhiatrii imeni S. S. Korsa-
    kova 67(8):1262.

SVYADOSHCH, A. M. (1971). Nevrozy i ikh lechenie [The neu-
    roses and their treatment], 2nd ed. Meditsina Publish-
    ing House, Moscow.

VOL'PERT, I. E. (1972). Psikhoterapiya [Psychotherapy].
    Meditsina Publishing House, Leningrad.

WORTIS, J. (1950). Soviet Psychiatry. Williams & Wilkins,
    Baltimore.

YAKOVLEVA, E. K. (1958). Patogenez i terapiya nevroza na-
    vyazchivykh sostoyanii i psikhastenii [Pathogenesis and
    theory of obsessive-compulsive neurosis and psychas-
    thenia]. Bekhterev Psychoneurological Research Insti-
    tute, Leningrad.

YUDIN, T. I. (1951). Ocherki istorii otechestvennoi psi-
    khiatrii [Essays on the history of Russian psychiatry].
    Medgiz, Moscow.

ZIFERSTEIN, I. (1965). Direct observations of psychotherapy
    in the U.S.S.R. In: Selected Lectures--Sixth Interna-
    tional Congress of Psychotherapy, ed. by M. Pines and
    T. Spoerri, S. Karger, Basel/New York.

ZIFERSTEIN, I. (1972). Group psychotherapy in the Soviet
    Union. Amer. J. Psychiat. 129(5):595-599.

ZURABASHVILI, A. D. (1963). Psikhoterapiya segodnya [Psycho-
    therapy today]. In: Aktual'nye voprosy psikhiatrii i
    nevropatologii [Current problems of psychiatry and
    neuropathology], ed. by G. V. Morozov, USSR Ministry
    of Health, pp. 363-368.

DRINKING PATTERNS AND ALCOHOLISM IN SOVIET AND

AMERICAN SOCIETIES: A MULTIDISCIPLINARY COMPARISON

Boris M. Segal

Russian Research Center
Harvard University
Cambridge, Massachusetts

It is well known that the development of alcoholism
is closely associated with many historical, cultural,
social, and psychological factors. Historical and social
conditions, economic and political structures, cultures
and traditions in American and Soviet societies are not
merely different; to a considerable extent, they are
antithetical. Do the prevalence of drinking and the
manifestation of the social and medical consequences of
alcoholism in both countries reflect these differences?

We shall attempt to analyze this interesting and
important cross-cultural problem from various perspectives,
although we shall not be able to examine all the details
within the limits imposed by the scope of a single article.

I.   DRINKING AND ALCOHOLISM IN SOVIET SOCIETY

Introductory Note

Drinking has always been a widespread phenomenon among
Northern and Slavic peoples. In particular, it is one of
the most deeply rooted Russian traditions. "What can be
said of our drunkenness! If you were to search the whole
world over, nowhere could you find such a vile, repulsive,
and terrible drunkenness as exists here in Russia...The
people...are exceptionally covetous of drinking, shameless,

This work was supported by a grant from the National
Institute on Alchohol Abuse and Alcoholism

181

and nearly mad, so that no matter how large a draught of
liquor you give them, they feel a divine and Sovereign
command to down it in a single gulp. And when they scrape
together some money and enter the infernal kabak (tavern),
they become totally demented and drink away all their
possessions and even the clothes on their backs" (1). So
wrote the Serbian priest Kryzhanich who settled in Russia
in the mid 17th century and who was subsequently exiled to
Siberia for his seditious pronouncements. (Such a response
by the government toward dissidents and critics is also an
old Russian tradition.)

    Loss of control in the drinking situation has always
been characteristic for Russia as well as for many other
Northern countries where "hard" alcoholic beverages are
used. In essence, the Russian Orthodox Church did not
totally limit this kind of drinking. Although the Church
theoretically condemned drunks, it did so in a rhetorical
way, since alcohol abuse was not infrequent among the
priests themselves. (A non-drinking pattern prevailed only
among certain groups, such as the Sectarians and the Old
Believers.) Until the Revolution, however, alcoholism was
widespread chiefly among workers and artisans in Russia.
Heavy drinking to the point of loss of control was limited
to ritual occasions; among peasants, it was usual only on
Church holidays, after the harvest, and on other festive
days. (True, on these days a single sober man could not be
found in the entire village, and drunks lined the streets.)
But a peasant who drank on working days was usually censured
as a drunkard and ne'er-do-well.

    Following the Revolution, a sizable number of peasants
migrated to the cities and now comprises a new and important
stratum of the urban society. The urban population has lost
the old peasant traditions and particularly the traditional
view of alcohol as a ritualistic element. This situation
was especially exacerbated after World War II, which swept
away millions of lives. From that time on, drinking has
been growing steadily. The majority of Russians now drink
regularly. Normally, they use alcohol on paydays. However,
a sizable portion of them drink on other days as well: on
weekends and any other days when they are able to obtain
money. Not only does regular, heavy drinking occur in all
the strata of the urban population, but it has recently also
developed among the rural population, which comprises over

40% of the total population. Intoxicated persons may now be found on any day of the week and at any time of day in rural as well as in urban areas. Heavy drinking is growing steadily among women and young people.

A. Drinking in Russia: Statistics, General Impact, and Relation to Family and to Some Types of Deviance

Although the official press formerly claimed that drunkenness and alcoholism, as the "remnants of capitalism in the people's consciousness," were rapidly vanishing from Soviet socialist society, it is now forced to admit the danger of these phenomena. At present, the mass media are sounding the alarm and reporting the prevalence of drunkenness among youth, the growing number of crimes committed under the influence of alcohol, and the deleterious effect of alcoholism on morality, family relations, and labor productivity.

However, like other data on Soviet society, published reports on the use of alcoholic beverages are incomplete and give no figures for the number of drinkers and alcoholics. According to official statistics, in pre-revolutionary Russia (1913), annual per capita consumption of 40% (80 proof) Vodka was 8.4 liters. As a result of passage of the "dry law," this figure fell sharply after the beginning of the war and the revolution. This law was partially rescinded in 1921 and completely abolished in 1925. Production of alcoholic beverages in state distilleries rose rapidly after repeal of the law. In 1925-1926 production amounted to 1.7 liters per capita; in 1927-1928 it was 3.6 liters; and in 1930-1931 the latter figure was doubled. State revenues from the sale of vodka reached 180 million rubles in 1926-1927 and were projected to amount to 360 million in 1930-1931. Subsequent statistical data were published irregularly, however, and those figures which were given are rather dubious. Data from the 1950s is available and indicates that 1.85 liters of 100% alcohol was consumed per capita annually. This figure is much lower than that for the rate of consumption in other developed countries (2). Later reports show a rise of consumption up to 4.7 liters of 100% alcohol.

National publication ceased in the 60s and 70s, but a number of indirect indications of an increase in this

figure were published. The data of the annual statistical
abstracts, Narodnoye khozyaistvo SSSR v 1962 godu, indicate
that the sale of alcoholic beverages grew 600% in the period
between 1940 and 1962 (3). The annual increase between
1956 and 1962 averaged 50%. The 1974 statistical abstracts
(Narodnoye khozyaistvo SSSR v 1973 godu), however, offer
other data (4). According to this new version, the sale of
alcoholic beverages was 283% in 1965 (taking 1940 as the
100% base figure), 439% in 1970, 422% in 1971, 501% in 1972,
and 531% in 1973. Even if these questionable figures are
accepted, it appears that the sale of alcoholic beverages
has increased by more than five times, while the population
of the Soviet Union within its present boundaries has
grown by only 50 million, or 25%, since 1940. According to
the sophisticated calculations made by the American economist V. Treml this year, the per capita consumption of
alcohol by persons of drinking age (15 and older) in the
Soviet Union is one of the highest in the world. The
Soviet Union shows the steepest rate of increase: 5.1%
annually per capita versus an average of 3.1% for 14
developed nations. Consumption of various state-distilled
alcoholic beverages totaled 1,500 million liters of 100%
alcohol annually (5). The consumption of illegal, home-
distilled "samogon" must also be taken into account.
According to Treml, "samogon" production equals 1 billion
liters of 100% alcohol per year. From this, Treml arrived
at a figure of 11.26 liters of 100% alcohol per capita
consumed by those over 15 years old. "Hard" liquor accounts
for 8.07 liters of this figure. Regions populated by Slavic
nationalities consume twice as much alcohol per capita as
Moslem regions (5).

    During the last ten to fifteen years, turnover taxes
on the sale of alcoholic beverages represented 10% to 12%
of all state revenues and over one-third of all taxes paid
by the population. The income from alcoholic beverages is
now higher than in pre-revolutionary Russia, whose budget
had been ironically dubbed "drunk." While taxes on spirits
supplied 5.4% of the national income in 1913, turnover tax
revenues and profits in the 1970s from the sale of alcoholic
beverages averaged some 21 to 23 billion rubles, or
approximately 7.3% of the national income (5).

    Reports made by the various republics on the fulfill-
ment of their economic plans list many food industry

products. At the end of this list there is usually a
section entitled "Other Food Industry Products." Most of
this section is devoted to listing alcoholic beverages,
which are thus "masked" by the heading. The reports of the
USSR Ministry of Trade for 1972 show that the sale of
products from this section totaled 30,922,000,000 rubles,
almost 30% of all food industry products sold (6). Our
supposition is supported by data from one republic, Latvia,
which for unknown reasons published information in 1972 on
the sale of alcoholic beverages. Alcoholic beverages
accounted for 29.3% of all food industry products sold
(7)*. Since alcohol consumption in Latvia is not higher
than in Russia, it is clear that the figure of some 30
billion rubles in fact represents the value of alcoholic
beverages sold. (Of course, in order to calculate the
profit from sales, the cost of alcoholic beverage production
must be subtracted from this sum.)

In the late 1960s, about 13% of the average Soviet
urban family budget reportedly was spent on alcohol (5).
We calculated that for the family of the Russian urban
drinker this figure amounts to approximately 50% of the
budget. Frequently, the alcoholic husband spends 100% of
his salary on alcohol and lives on his spouse's income.
Many heavy drinkers purchase alcoholic beverages with
supplementary incomes they conceal from their families.

According to Urlanis, a prominent Soviet demographer,
the government's economic losses from drunkenness exceed
its income from the sale of alcoholic beverages (8). In
other words, these losses are not less than 25 to 30
billion rubles (5).

As we noted above, Soviet mass media and educational
literature have admitted in recent years the great harm of
drunkenness to society. According to various publications,
approximately half of all fatal traffic accidents involve
drunken drivers and three-fourths involve drunken pedestrians (9, 10). Tkachevsky and other authors have noted that
90% to 95% of all incidents of hooliganism are committed by

---

* This is more than the population bought in meat, fish,
fowl, sausage, eggs, butter, and all other fats combined,
and constitutes 14.5% of all consumer goods.

persons in an intoxicated state (11, 12, 13). Alcoholics
are much more frequently punished, laid off, and demoted.
Stealing is also closely associated with drunkenness (11,
12, 13), since many Russian alcoholics resort to stealing
to finance their drinking. (Prices of alcoholic beverages
are relatively high in relation to the low income of the
Soviet citizen; for example, the average price of vodka is
7 to 8 rubles per liter, while the average income of a Soviet
worker or office employee, according to official data, is
only 134.9 rubles per month.) According to data in
Alcoholism—The Road to Crime (13), 66.5% of murders and
68.6% of rapes are committed in an intoxicated state. We
estimated that various kinds of violations were committed
by 70% of the 1703 alcoholics we surveyed (14). A
forensic-psychiatric commission of experts reported that
83% of the persons who had committed violations in a
state of drunkenness were alcoholics (15).

It has been reported (16-18) that labor productivity after
a weekend falls by at least 30% as a consequence of
drunkenness, which is also the cause for many accidents at
work (16,17). Of the 1703 alcoholics we surveyed, 98%
periodically reported to work in an intoxicated state (14).
Our data shows that alchoholics had four times as many
violations of social, economic, and working conditions as
nonalcoholics, and three times as many divorces. 45% of
the male alcoholics and 59% of the female alcoholics
surveyed were divorced (14). It has also been reported
that 40% to 50% of all divorces were associated with
alcohol abuse by one of the spouses (19). Emotional
disorders, juvenile delinquency, and a disposition to
early alcohol use occur with a high frequency among children
who grow up in an atmosphere of drunken scandals, swearing,
and fighting (10, 12, 14, 16, 17).

Official data on the incidence of physical complication
of an alcoholic etiology have not been published, but there
are many reports dealing with the role of alcoholic
intoxication in the origin of cirrhosis of the liver,
pancreatitis, cardiovascular disorders, ulcerous diseases
of the stomach and duodenum, etc.

For instance, it has been reported (20) that among
2,736 survivors, heart and vessel disorders occurred before

the onset of alcoholism in 1.3% of all cases, gastrointestinal diseases in 1.1% of the cases, and respiratory
diseases in 1.7% of the cases. After the onset of
alcoholism, these rates comprised, respectively, 32.4%,
22.8% and 6.4% of the cases, i.e., they increased 25, 20
and 4 times. Since all the patients were relatively
young, the author considered these somatic disorders the
consequence of alcoholism.

Statistical information on the total number of
alcoholics in the Soviet Union is also unavailable.
Officials from the Soviet Ministry of Health usually give
evasive answers to questions on this topic and sometimes,
to the most insistent foreign visitors, quote the figure
of 6 alcoholics per 1,000 population. The data presented
below shows that psychiatric institutions' reports on the
number of "registered" alcoholics are used in arriving
at this figure.

A comparison of these reports makes apparent a sharp
increase in incidence. Thus, for Moscow, the number of
registered alcoholics was 3.1 per 10,000 population in
1946, 5.5 in 1950, 5.6 in 1958, and 7.4 in 1959.
Alcoholics registered in psychiatric dispensaries in the
RSFSR in these years made up roughly 25% of all patients
(21). In 1954, alcoholics accounted for 13.5% of all
admissions to mental hospitals, and in 1959, 40% (21).

If we take into account the fact that during this
period there were approximately 1,900,000 "registered"
psychiatric patients in the Soviet Union, we would expect,
according to our calculations, 250,000 "registered"
alcoholics. But already in 1968, figures on the prevalence
of alcoholism, based on data gathered during visits to a
number of urban dispensaries, proved to be 10 (!) times
higher: an average of 8 per 1,000 of the population (22).
If this figure is extrapolated for the entire population
of urban areas, there were approximately 1,120,000
alcoholics in cities at that time.

Fewer alcoholics are "registered" in predominantly
rural areas. According to some data, there are 5.4
alcoholics per 1,000 of the population (23). We must
certainly take into account that rural areas have very
poor psychiatric care services: there is usually one

psychiatric dispensary in a region of several million
inhabitants. Nevertheless, an extrapolation would
yield the figure of approximately 570,000 alcoholics
in rural areas. Thus, the total number of registered
alcoholics in psychiatric dispensaries in the Soviet
Union should be between 1,500,000 and 1,700,000, and
in the RSFSR (the Russian Federation) between 800,000 and
1 million.

However, as even some Soviet authors admit, the
"registered" number does not reflect the true extent of
alcoholism (21-24). A comparison of the incidence in
various provinces of the RSFSR that have a fairly even
distribution of drunkenness makes it apparent that the
number of registered alcoholics fluctuates between 0.1%
and 74.3% of the total number of registered patients
(21). Soviet authors correctly explain this discrepancy
as arising from the variations in the activity of regional
dispensaries: some dispensaries treat alcoholism more
intensively, while others shun this thankless work. It
is for this reason that the latter figure, 74% to 75%,
is more accurate than the average rate of 25%. Estimates
show that this figure yields 26 alcoholics per 1,000
persons. Thus, in 1973 there should have been 6,500,000
alcoholics in the Soviet Union and 3,500,000 in the
RSFSR.

True, we did not take into consideration regional
differences: there is less alcoholism in other republics
than in the RSFSR. On the other hand, we must keep in
mind that, particularly in the provinces, dispensaries
register only those cases of alcoholism that are acute
and accompanied by severe disruption of social relations,
lengthy hard-liquor drunkenness, and psychoses (the third
stage, according to my classification) (14). The majority
of alcoholics, especially women, young people, and members
of the middle and upper classes, usually avoid turning
to the psychiatric dispensary.

Thus, in order to establish the real incidence of
drinking and alcoholism, we conducted an epidemiological
study of the population. Between 1965 and 1972, we
surveyed 12,475 people, of whom 5,383 were from the
Russian Federation (RSFSR). The survey was conducted in
the form of a questionnaire investigating the health of

the population. Various social, professional, and ethnic
groups in urban and rural areas of a number of Soviet
republics were studied. In order to obtain more reliable
results, we investigated a variety of social and age
groups in rural and urban societies and extrapolated the
resulting data for corresponding groups in the total
population. Only after this did we carry out our final
evaluation.

Although I am convinced that alcoholism is a multidimensional process, we felt that the goals of this study
were better served by a unidimensional model. It was
used as the model for the development of alcoholism which
I proposed in 1967 (14). This model is based on the
principle of the dynamic craving for alcohol and different forms of addiction; social, psychological, and
medical criteria were used as supplementary factors (see
below, "Criteria").

In this article, I will briefly present data on only
the largest Soviet republic - the Russian Federation (the
RSFSR), which may be called "Russia" in the narrower
sense of the word. This republic has a population of
132.9 million out of the total Soviet population of
250.8 million (1973). The majority of the population is
of Russian nationality (122.8 million). Many of the
largest Soviet industrial and cultural centers are
located in the RSFSR.

The Russian Federation proved to have the highest
incidence of drinking and alcoholism: according to our
calculations, there were 86 million drinkers (90.7% of
the population over 15) and 10.4 million alcoholics or
problem drinkers (11% of the population over 15, or 13%
of the population over 21). In second place came two
Slavic Republics, Belorussia and the Ukraine, followed by
the Baltic Republics: Estonia, Latvia, and Lithuania.
Less than half the alcoholics may be included in the
category of addictive alcoholics ("drug dependence--
alcohol type"), or, according to my scheme, in the
classification of the second and third stage of
alcoholism.

Among drinkers, 7.5% consume alcoholic beverages
systematically, many times a month, and usually have five
or more drinks each time. They are frequently drunk and
lose control over the amount of alcohol they consume.
They do not, however, manifest other clinical and social
features of alcoholism. Thus, it is possible to classify
this group as "pre-alcoholic." This group may be combined
with alcoholics (problem drinkers) in the category of
"heavy drinkers." Together, both these groups comprise
18.5% of the population over 15.

32% of all children between the ages of 8 and 15 use
alcoholic beverages (more than one drink in the past year,
usually in the form of wine or beer). 5.5% of children
drink regularly during holidays. The survey revealed that
46% of 15 year-olds drink, 67% of 16 year-olds, 71% of 17
year-olds, 86% of 18 year-olds, and 95% of 21 year-olds.
Corresponding data for persons of Russian nationality,
who make up 92.8% of the total population of the RSFSR,
are even higher.

94.6% of Russians over 15 years of age drink, 11.6%
are alcoholics, and 19% are heavy drinkers. Among children
of Russian nationality and between the ages of 10 and 15,
34.4% drink occasionally; i.e., not less than one drink
in the past year (53.8% boys and 15.2% girls) and 6%
drink regularly on holidays. In regions of high wine
consumption (the Caucasus and Moldavia), a discrepancy
was noted between the relatively high incidence of
drinking and the relatively low incidence of alcoholism.
The lowest figures for drinking and alcoholism were
found in the Central Asian republics, whose population
consists primarily of Moslems, and among Jews. The
figures for these regions are responsible for making the
general figures for the Soviet Union lower than those
for the RSFSR.

From a social point of view, the highest incidence of
alcoholism is found among male urban blue-collar workers
and among workers in the services sphere who have a
supplementary income. Alcoholism among white-collar
workers, the intelligentsia, and the establishment is
usually more covert and controlled. The ratio of male to
female alcoholics is 8.5:1.

B. Russian Drinking Behavior

Vodka is the typical "hard" liquor in the Russian
drinking pattern. However, other types of "hard" liquor
such as cognac (although this is confined to the more
affluent and cultured circles) is also willingly consumed.
Blue-collar workers, artisans, and peasants drink "samogon"
in addition to these, and, when possible, rectified spirit.
The latter can only be obtained illegally, since it is not
available on the market. The stronger the alcoholic
beverage, the greater the respect it inspires. In addition
to all these varieties, alcoholics also drink such
substitutes as Eau-de-Cologne, drugs in spirit, and
industrial spirits (which often produce poisoning).

Beer is popular in Russia, although it is often used
as a chaser to strengthen the effect of vodka. In the
Slavic and Baltic regions, wines are consumed less frequently
than vodka and are used chiefly by women. Here the population prefers fortified wines, such as port, to grape wines.
Grape wines are primarily drunk in the southern regions:
in the Caucasus and in Moldavia.

Alcoholic beverages are an integral part of any form
of social relations and contacts: entertaining guests, on
holidays, funerals, births, marriages, sexual relations,
etc. Drinking is not only ritualistic, it is also utilitarian, since it is used for consolidating business contracts,
attaining social success, and establishing good relations
with supervisors.

It is a characteristic practice to coerce guests to
drink. The host and guests persistently offer each other
drinks and are highly insulted by any refusal. Such an
action is interpreted as a lack of respect for the person
offering a drink. This custom is a remnant of the old
Russian, widespread patriarchal hospitality. A capacity
for great quantities has long been considered a mark of
true virility, valor, and breadth of character and earns
the respect of the entire company. Although the "duels" -
sometimes fatal - have vanished almost entirely, an
unspoken competition in drinking persists as before. Not
only nondrinkers but even persons with a low drinking
capacity are subjected to censure and ridicule. The urge for
drunkenness per se often predominates over hedonistic aims,

over the desire to achieve a moderate euphoria. Rarely do men stop with the "necessary dose," that which produces euphoria without distinct behavioral disturbances; often they continue drinking until they lose control over the amount of alcohol consumed, to the point of considerable psychic and motor symptoms of intoxication. Wine and vodka are never diluted with water and are rarely drunk slowly in small doses. The male pattern consists of drinking alcohol by the glass, in a single draught followed by a light appetizer. Recently even women have adopted this custom. Although Soviet law does not view drunkenness as a condition extenuating guilt in crime, national consciousness claims that "the guilt lies with the vodka, not the man." Thus, the traditional Russian drinking pattern among Soviet workers and peasants has now been modified by almost total permissiveness.

As we noted above, the intelligentsia and white-collar workers hold more moderate attitudes toward drinking. Mixed and negative views are more often observed among Moslems and Jews.

All these features characterize the national customs observed by the majority of the population in the central, eastern, western, and northern regions of the country. Although positive attitudes toward drinking also predominate in the southern, mainly grape-wine consuming regions, the drinking patterns here are slightly different. Wine is the principal alcoholic beverage, and it is drunk regularly. It is not used solely for ritualistic and utilitarian purposes, however, but also as a form of nutrition and is drunk with meals. This circumstance in part accounts for a lower rate of alcoholism in the southern regions. Here, as in the Russian Republic, refusal to accept a drink is viewed as an insult to the host, who expresses his hospitality by pressing as much alcohol on his guest as possible. However, grossly incorrect drinking behavior is much more severely condemned than in the RSFSR. With the adoption of Russian customs in these regions, strong liquors such as cognac, vodka, and grape "samogon" (the Georgian "Chacha") have begun to be consumed more frequently. Consequently, alcoholism has begun to increase among the local populations.

C. Soviet Data on the Etiology of Alcoholism

For a long time Soviet authors emphatically fixed
the causes of drinking in the "survivals of capitalism in
the people's consciousness" and in "bad customs." They
considered alcoholism the result of conditioned (extero-
ceptive and interoceptive) reflex mechanisms (9, 16, 17,
25). Physiological experiments, particularly on dogs,
were based on Pavlovian technique (9). Almost no
investigations were made into other possible etiological
factors, and psychological causes of drinking were not
examined. This situation has only recently begun to
change. Research, especially using electrophysiological
and biochemical methods, has increased. Individual
sociological and genetic studies have also begun to appear.
Various concepts of the etiology of alcoholism have been
analyzed, and the present author in particular dealt with
this topic (14). Our analysis showed no apparent
differences in the social, economic, and educational backgrounds of alcoholics (before the onset of alcoholism) and
social drinkers.

The influence of sociopsychological factors such as
drinking patterns, family attitudes, and environment proved
very clear. In 70% of the cases, the alcoholics' parents
tolerated drunkenness, and in 10% of the cases, they even
accepted heavy drinking. Even more striking data were
obtained in a study of "friends" (referent groups), among
whom heavy drinking was the norm in 53% of the cases, and
"moderate" drinking in 43%. The negative influence of
"friends" was most evident among teenage drinkers.

The study showed that a pre-alcoholic state
accompanied by expressed neurotic and psychopathic
symptoms was present in 19.8% to 26.1% of the cases (in
various groups). Most of the remaining patients were in the
category of the so-called "persons of external norm"
(Luxenburger). The only danger which exists for these
persons is the "danger of disintegration" under stress.
"True" neurotics, for instance, those with obvious
obsessivephobic syndromes, become alcoholics relatively
rarely. Brain injuries magnified the craving for alcohol
($p < 0.01$). Thirty-three percent of all cases sought the
tranquilizing effect of alcohol, and 20% sought stimulating
and euphoric effects (14, 26).

More than half the cases (52.5%) revealed an "unhappy childhood" (lack of a parent, etc.). Such factors as a domineering mother and oral habits did not correlate with the rapid start of alcoholism. However, early weaning accompanied by rapid development of physical dependency (secondary pathologic craving for alcohol) was found to be significant.

Suppressed aggressive and destructive impulses, on the one hand, and such traits as dependence and introversion, on the other, played an important role. Psychological tests, e.g., the MMPI and TAT,* also revealed the presence of a low tolerance to frustration, a sense of guilt, anxiety and depression, masochistic-type behavior, hostility and anger, maladjustment, and sexual problems. All our patients refused for many years to recognize the fact that they were alcoholics and used the defensive mechanisms of denial, rationalization, and projection of blame to their spouses or other persons. We emphasized, however, that many of these characteristics, such as anxiety, sense of guilt, depression, are the consequence rather than the cause of alcoholism and are manifested only in the withdrawal period (14, 26).

We observed a premorbid failure of the autonomic and endocrine systems in only 13.5% of the cases. These insufficiencies were present twice as often in patients with an early history of alcoholism as in patients with a late development of the disease. In addition, the possibility of subtle and latent neurohumoral deviations must be considered; verification of their existence, however, requires laboratory testing which, understandably, is not carried out before the onset of alcoholism.

Experiments with rats have shown that a link exists between the craving for alcohol and the functional state of the hypothalamic system (27, 28). After the "punishment system" was stimulated, a craving for alcohol was initiated. Alcohol consumption either decreased or ceased entirely when the "reinforcement system" was stimulated and self-stimulated and when reactions of a food-consuming or sexual nature were observed. Voluntary consumption of alcohol and minor tranquilizers raised the threshold of irritation in the "punishment system" and weakened defensive responses.

Despite the prevailing official views, in 1967 the

---

*Minnesota Multiphasic Personality Inventory
and Thematic Apperception Test

present writer, on the basis of epidemiological, clinical, psychological, and physiological studies, expressed his opinion that social drinking becomes widespread when a society cannot satisfy the individual's needs, especially the need for a meaningful existence, and when the prevailing attitude toward alcohol abuse is permissive (14). At the same time I concluded that emotional deprivations in childhood and certain personality peculiarities play an important role in the development of heavy drinking beyond the limits proscribed by a given society (but note that only some of the cases of personality peculiarities can be qualified as true neurotics and psychopaths (14). My conclusions differed little from those which Western psychiatrists reached simultaneously, but they were unusual and controversial in the Soviet Union and were viewed as a "concession to reactionary psychoanalysis."

My colleagues and I noted that during the period of deprivation the serotonin level drops in the blood and the norepinephrine level decreases in the urine, the activity of the hypophysial-adrenal system and the thyroid gland is suppressed, and some other biochemical and autonomic disorders take place which attest to the disruption of adaptive and homeostatic functions (14, 28). Our clinical, experimental, and laboratory data permitted us to formulate the concept of alcohol disorders as resulting from the dysfunction of the limbico-reticulo-hypothalamic structures (14, 28). (See also the section "Research.")

D. Criteria for the Diagnosis of Alcoholism

In the past, the concept of chronic alcoholism elaborated by Magnus Huss in 1849 and supplemented by some German and Russian psychiatrists was widely used by Soviet writers. Soviet handbooks described chronic alcoholism as the excessive use of alcoholic beverages that produces changes in the nervous system and in the internal organs; the "habit" or "craving for alcohol" were sometimes noted, but only as secondary features (Gurevich, Gilyarovsky, Popov, Strelchuk) (9, 25, 29-31). The evolution of these opinions was promoted by two separate influences. On the one hand, these were the views of the Soviet psychiatrist Zhislin who in 1929 described the alcohol abstinence syndrome ("sindrom pokhmel'is"), although his work remained unknown in the West (32). On the other hand, the impact of new Western concepts of alcohol craving and addiction contributed to modifications in views on chronic alcoholism.

In 1967 we proposed the following definition: "Alcoholism
is a disease caused by systematic alcohol abuse, characterized by a pathologic craving for alcohol, which results in
psychological and physical disorders and disruptions of
the individual's social relations" (14).

I believe that Jellinek's concept of loss of control
over the consumption of alcohol calls for a more precise
definition. As we noted above, severe intoxication, which
externally resembles this symptom, is frequent among
Russian nonalcoholic drinkers. However, this form of alcohol
abuse is basically determined by social and psychological
factors and, if necessary, can be controlled. This symptom
is considerably more manifest among alcoholics. It is
basically pathological and does not lend itself to social
and psychological control. According to my classification,
the first phase of alcoholism is marked by excessive drinking
that leads to problems in health and interpersonal relationships. Many of these reveal signs of the loss of control
over the use of alcohol and the psychological craving for
alcohol. However, this phase may be basically labelled the
"nonaddictive alcoholism." As can be seen from our
definition, this phase resembles the "nonaddictive pathological drinking" described by Strauss and McCarthy. It
differs from the latter in that it includes the criterion
of loss of control over drinking. (As we noted above, the
Russian pathological nonaddictive drinker seeks a "peak"
effect in intoxication rather than the "plateau" which his
American counterpart strives for.) Alcoholics in this phase
may also be termed "problem drinkers."

The second stage is characterized by a clear withdrawal
syndrome with expressed physical dependence (addiction),
considerable disruption of social and family relations, and
somatic disorders. All the symptoms of an altered reaction
toward alcohol (changes of tolerance, type of intoxication,
system of drinking, etc.) are clearly manifested in this
phase. The third stage is distinguished by periodic bouts
of heavy drinking and psychoses (14). Both of these phases
may be labelled "addictive alcoholism" or "drug dependence--
alcohol type."

At present, all Soviet works emphasize the progressive
character of alcoholism. Most authors describe three
stages (phases) of this disease.

E. Methods of Social Prevention and Medical Measures

"Societies of sobriety" existed in prerevolutionary Russia, but the government took a minimal part in preventing drunkenness. During the first years of the Revolution, alcoholism was proclaimed a social disease. Dispensaries (mental health centers) were open with the primary goal of carrying on preventive work among the population. At the same time, the development of mental hygiene was initiated and narcological consultation rooms and centers were organized for the treatment of alcoholics and the dissemination of antialcohol propaganda. However, this progressive system was not successfully carried through. Mental hygiene was forbidden in Stalin's time, and the dispensaries were transformed into ordinary out-patient clinics. According to the ruling thesis, the land of "triumphant socialism" had already almost totally liquidated such survivals of the past as alcoholism. It has now become apparent, however, that this problem not only has not been solved but has assumed threatening proportions. The government and officials in the health services now understand the dangerous consequences of the growth of drunkenness and alcoholism and have already under-taken and continue to undertake urgent countermeasures.

A broad campaign has been initiated against "alcoholic prejudices" and "bad traditions." Doctors, scientists, educators, and representatives of the government and police now lecture to the people on the harm of alcohol and the dangerous medical and social consequences of drunkenness. Orders have been issued to local government agencies to control all these measures. The government, however, fear-ful of any nongovernment organizations, rejects proposals to revive the prerevolutionary "Societies of Sobriety" or to create an organization along the lines of Alcoholics Anonymous.

The price of vodka has been raised many times (during Khrushchev's administration and again in 1970 and 1973) with the aim of curtailing consumption. New resolutions have been passed on intensifying the campaign against home-brewing and limiting the hours of retail sale of alcoholic beverages. The Supreme Soviet issued a decree on stepping up the

campaign against hooliganism and drunkenness in public
places. The government also decided to limit production
of vodka in favor of increased production of wine and beer.
The police constantly receive orders to crack down on the
practice of home-brewing. In 1974 the RSFSR Supreme Soviet
ratified a decree proposing the creation of a system of
institutions within the Ministry of Internal Affairs (the
police) for the compulsory treatment and vocational
reeducation of "persistent drunks" and alcoholics manifesting antisocial behavior (33).

In the 1940s and 1950s alcoholics were not considered
"real patients" and the Ministry of Health denied hospitalization to nonpsychotic alcoholics. Relatives of alcoholics
would spend months in unsuccessful appeals to have these
patients, the victims of discrimination, admitted to treatment. The situation has now improved in this respect. Over
the course of several years, a system of medical care for
alcoholics has been developed and is being perfected under
the auspices of the Ministry of Health. This system
comprises, first, special "narcological offices" associated
with psychiatric dispensaries (mental health centers) and
health service units in large factories and, second,
alcoholic departments at psychiatric hospitals (14, 25, 34,
41, 45, 46). These institutions are well organized in the
largest cities (Moscow, Leningrad, Kiev). They are inter-
connected in order to ensure continuity of treatment,
provide care after completion of the basic course of
treatment, contact the patient's family and supervisors,
and sometimes assist the patient in solving urgent social
and family problems. The situation is different, however,
in smaller cities and in rural areas, which still account
for 65% of the total population. Here the system of
community mental health centers exists only on paper.
Service is especially inadequate in rural areas, where 40%
of the total population now lives.

Treatment of the first stage of alcoholism consists of
detoxification and the prescribing of tranquilizers and
vitamins. The second stage is treated through antabuse
treatment and conditioned-reflex therapy with aversive drugs
Soviet authors have proposed a number of new variants of
medication (Lycopodium selago as a potent aversive drug,

sodium thiosulfatum, dithiols, etc.) (9, 14, 25, 34-36).
Psychotherapy is used less frequently, mainly because of
the lack of time and qualified specialists. When
psychotherapy is used, it is conducted in the form of short-
term therapy, individual and group "rational psychotherapy"
(persuasion) and suggestion (hypnosis) (9, 14, 25, 34-38,
40 - 45). Recently, autogenic training has come into
practice, and especially our method of combining relaxation
with suggestion and autosuggestion (14, 39).

What is the result of all these efforts? It must be
noted, first of all, that the measures the government has
undertaken are half-measures and are inconsistently applied.
This is specifically related to the fact that the government
has a vested economic interest in the sale of alcoholic
beverages. On the other hand, in any bureaucratic system
even the best resolutions may not be realized. Thus, the
decision to wage a campaign against public drunkenness has
not been carried out. Many drunks can still be seen on the
city streets, especially in the outskirts. The campaign
against home-brewing has also been ineffective: the
number of people who engage in this activity is very great,
and the police can always be bribed. As in other countries
that have resorted to raising the price of liquor, the price
hike on vodka has had little effect on the level of
consumption. Lectures and "antialcoholic" propaganda usually
produce an ironic response among people who have positive
drinking attitudes. Corresponding educational measures
among children are lacking (see below). While enterprises
and social organizations often try to influence alcoholics
by moralizing and punishing, this too is, as a rule,
ineffective.

The prevention system is also imperfect. It exists
in only some parts of major cities and is usually predominantly pro forma. The great deficiency of the
organization of alcoholic treatment is that the entire
burden of work is assumed by doctors and nurses, who are
in short supply. There are no social workers in the
Soviet Union. Only the most serious forms of alcoholism,
with disruption of social functions, are admitted to treatment. After-care is not always provided. Psychiatrists
and physicians treat alcoholics reluctantly.

Evaluating the effectiveness of treatment is a very
complex problem and depends on many factors: selection of
patients, their attitude toward therapy and toward the
therapist, the therapist's personality, the chosen method,
its duration, follow-up care, etc. The very wide range of
the evaluation of the effectiveness of treatment is therefore not accidental. According to various Soviet authors,
a treatment is considered good if it produces remissions
lasting well over a year, occurring in between 5.4% and
82.5% of all cases (9, 14, 25, 34-36, 40-45). The best
results—good remissions exceeding 30%-60% of all cases—are
obtained when a combination of detoxifying therapy, antabuse
therapy, and psychotherapy is used. Reviewing these data,
we may conclude that the average duration of remissions
after treatment is relatively brief. Our data shows that
in most cases it fluctuates between 10.4 and 15 months (14).
Relapses occurred before this time in roughly one-third of
the cases, and "good" results, with abstinence lasting more
than a year, occurred in approximately the same proportion
of cases. The majority of Soviet writers accord special
significance to the so-called clinical factors in obtaining
good results: the alcoholic stage, deterioration, organic
symptoms, etc. This hypothesis, however, was not confirmed
by our investigation (14). Reports on the role of social
and psychological factors have appeared only in recent years.

F. Research

Several research departments conduct studies in the
area of alcoholism in the larger cities (Moscow, Leningrad,
Kiev). One of the persistent problems that faces all types
of Soviet research is the difficulty of obtaining foreign
scientific information. It is also extremely difficult for
a Soviet scientist to publish his work abroad. While a
number of articles, monographs, and dissertations has been
published, it is still inadequate. The usual publication
consists of a collection of short articles, some meriting
attention, though not all on a very high level (13, 36,
40-45). The great majority of works attempt to establish
correlations between various clinical syndromes or phases
of alcoholism and biochemical or electrophysiological
indicators. Some books and articles describe the methods
of treatment used in the Soviet Union and the organization
of medical services (34, 35, 41, 45). The Western reader

would certainly benefit from an acquaintance with this experience of Russian psychiatrists. However, only a very few substantial theoretical works have been devoted to alcoholism. Some of them present an insufficiently consistent attempt to modernize the traditional Soviet approach to alcoholism, which is based on the conditioned reflex theory, with haphazardly and tendentiously chosen references to contemporary Western studies (25). Others contain only clinical (descriptive) material, and their theoretical sections are not based on the authors' own research but are purely speculative (46).

Almost none of the laboratories deal exclusively with the scientific problem of alcoholism. Laboratories take on research on alcoholism in addition to their basic, regular programs. Their work is hampered by outdated equipment and a shortage of experienced personnel.

As we mentioned above, social and psychological aspects of the problem have begun to be analyzed only recently. The lag in this area is related to the fact that the alcoholism problem does not carry enough prestige and that the government does not allot sufficient revenues for this purpose. Moreover, there is not a single center which could coordinate research activity. Sociological investigations represent a dangerous topic for Party leadership, and ideological control over research is still strongly maintained.

As all of this makes apparent, there is on the whole very little success in the areas of prevention, treatment, and research, and the problem of alcoholism remains a veritable disaster area in both the social and the medical sense.

II. DRINKING AND ALCOHOLISM IN THE UNITED STATES

COMPARED TO THE USSR

A. A Comparison of Statistical Data

Drunkenness and alcoholism also represent very serious problems in the United States. Although U. S. statistics for this area are more extensive than in the Soviet Union, even they are not exhaustive. Below we will present such

American figures as may be compared to the corresponding
Soviet rates.

Alcohol consumption is increasing in the United States,
although not as rapidly as in the Soviet Union, where the
growth rate is the highest in the world. Consumption of
alcohol in the United States increased by 26% during the
period between 1960 and 1970. While the United States
showed a 90% increase in per capita alcohol consumption
between 1950 and 1973, the increase in the Soviet Union was
at least 500% (4, 47). According to 1973 statistics, 10.6
liters of 100% alcohol were consumed per person by those
over 15 years of age in the United States (48), a figure
very close to the Soviet one. Both of these figures fall
below the levels of alcohol consumption in such "wine"
countries as France, Portugal, and Spain. At the same time,
however, the Soviet Union and the United States are among
the 10 countries with the highest level of consumption of
alcoholic beverages. But more important than this is the
fact that both countries occupy first place in the world in
the consumption of distilled spirits. Soviets consume
almost twice as much as Americans (8.07 liters and 4.25
liters of 100% alcohol respectively). A national survey of
drinking conducted in the continental United States in
1964-1965 showed that of 2746 individuals over 21 years old
68% drank at least once a year. Only 12% of the respondents
were classified as "heavy drinkers" (i.e., people who drink
nearly every day and at least weekly had five or more drinks
at any one time) (43-51). According to Calahan's scoring
procedures, 9% of the individuals in the sample (15% of the
men and 4% of the women) had scores which would seem to
indicate problem drinking (51). All these figures are
significantly lower than the corresponding figures for the
Russian survey. A survey conducted in South Carolina in
1965 showed that 26% of the males and 17% of the females
tried alcoholic beverages at the age of 13 or younger (52).
In 1971, the Georgia Department of Public Health conducted
a survey of 42,000 students from urban and rural schools
(53). Of the students surveyed, 36.5% between the ages of
12 and 18 used alcohol; at the age of 12, 18.9% used alcohol
at the age of 13, 23.8%; 14, 30.5%; 15, 39.3%; 16, 46.2%;
17, 52.8%; 18, 55.4%. A comparison of these figures with
corresponding Russian figures reveals that the latter are
not only higher but show a sharp increase at the age of 16

(the legal drinking age in the Soviet Union) and another
sharp rise at the time of commencing work. Social class,
age, sex, ethnicity, religious background, and urban or
rural residence also influenced adolescent drinking in both
countries. More young people than old people drink in both
societies: in the Soviet Union 95% of the people over 21
and in the United States 82% of college graduates. Both
these figures are above the average figures for both
populations. (See below: "Age and Sex Factors.")

According to data of the NIAAA and the NCA, about 100
million Americans drink (i.e., 62.5% of the population over
15) and 9 million are alcoholics or problem drinkers (5.6%
of the population over 15).* Although these figures are
very high, they are approximately 33% to 50% lower than the
corresponding figures for the Soviet Union, especially for
the Russian regions. Both countries reveal a tendency
toward a rise in the number of drinkers and toward an increasing proportion of alcoholics among them (in the period
between 1940 and 1953 the number of alcoholics in the United
States rose by 44%; in 1952 they made up 1% of the adult
population, and in 1955, 4.4%).

Major American industrial firms report that an alcoholic
loses 22 more working days per year than his nonalcoholic
counterpart and suffers twice as many accidents. The NIMH
recently estimated losses due to alcohol abuse at 15
billion dollars annually (54). Inasmuch as the rate of
alcoholism among employees is higher in the Soviet Union,
these losses must be all the greater here. As we noted
above, Soviet losses due to alcohol abuse reach a minimum
of 25 to 30 billion rubles annually, and probably even more.

Human losses and total cost to the nation and families
in both countries defy calculation. The National Safety
Council reported that in the United States about 800,000
highway accidents and 28,000 deaths (i.e., 50% of all fatal
accidents) each year result from the intoxication of drivers

---

*At present, the figure of 10 million problem drinkers
is also cited. However, the number of alcohol addicts is
figured apparently in the range of 5-6 million.

and pedestrians. Alcoholism, rather than social drinking, is responsible for the majority of these accidents. Information on the general number of traffic accidents in the Soviet Union is not available. In view of the fact that there are fewer automobiles in the Soviet Union, these figures may be lower than in the United States, but the proportion of accidents connected with alcohol is not lower in the Soviet Union (about 50% to 75% of all fatal accidents) (8, 9). In addition, in the RSFSR as many as 10,000 people freeze to death each winter by falling down outdoors while drunk (55).

FBI reports indicate that public intoxication accounts for one-third of all arrests each year; in half of all murders either the killer or the victim was drinking. In some states, California for example, this figure is more than half of all arrests (56). According to other figures, alcohol is involved in 31% to 64% of all homicides, 70% of all physical assault crimes, 50% of all shootings and other forms of assault, and 11% to 60% of all suicides (57-59). The National Council on Alcoholism reports that 24% of alcoholic deaths are violent. Soviet data on this issue are selective. However, the proportion of violations and crimes associated with alcohol is apparently even higher in the Soviet Union. Above we cited data to the effect that two-thirds of all murders, 68.8% of all rapes, and 90% to 95% of all cases of hooliganism are connected with drunkenness (11-15). The last figure reflects the more aggressive type of drinking behavior which is found in Russia.

The number of disrupted family relations (divorces) connected with alcohol abuse is roughly identical for both countries (not less than 40% to 50% of all cases). Disruption of family and social life often leads to severe maladjustment in children and contributes to present and future delinquency (in the United States, 30% to 40% of all delinquent youths come from alcoholic homes), school dropouts crime, neurosis, alcoholism, inadequate personality, etc. (12-17, 60-69). According to Bailey and Leach (63), each alcoholic directly affects four to five other people.

Both societies have an analogous incidence of various diseases caused by alcoholism. Although the information on this topic is far from complete, it is possible to state

that alcoholism ranks among the major health hazards, along
with cancer, mental illness and heart disease. The role of
alcohol in morbidity is significant. It has been established
that alcoholism leads to certain forms of hepatitis,
gastritis, certain hematological disorders, peripheral
neuropathy, cerebral atrophy, cardio-vascular and nutritional
disorders, and probably some forms of cancer.* The role of
alcoholism in cirrhosis is well known. Alcoholism is one of
the most frequent causes of various mental disorders. In
the United States and in the Soviet Union, about 40% to 50%
of all patients admitted to state mental hospitals suffer
from alcoholism. The average annual death rate of American
alcoholics—according to the NCA—was two and one-half times
the normal death rate, and the life expectancy of an alcoholic
is some 12 years less than normal. Soviet sources report
that the life expectancy of alcoholics is 15 years below
that for nonalcoholics (25).

B. Attitudes Toward Drinking Among Different Cultural and
Social Groups in American and Soviet Societies

Both in the United States and in the Soviet Union,
drinking and alcoholism is unevenly distributed among various
ethnic, social, and professional groups. As has been mentioned above, the greatest prevalence in the Soviet Union is
found in the northern, eastern, and central regions of the
Russian Republic, and in the other Slavic and Baltic
Republics. Despite population migration these differences
are more persistent in the Soviet Union than in the United
States, where the influence of historical and ethnic factors
is less long-term and concrete for different regions.
(Individual ethnic and religious groups do not occupy such
significant areas of the United States.) Past reports
indicate that the highest proportion of drinkers occurs in

---

*As an example, we would like to offer the data of Pell
and D'Alonzo (64), who in their study of 76,687 cases found
the following relationship between prevalence of chronic
disease among problem drinkers and the control group: the
ratio for hypertension in problem drinkers as compared to
the control group was 2.3:1; for coronary heart disease,
1.3:1; for cerebrovascular disease, 2.0:1; for cirrhosis of
the liver, 29.0:1; for stomach ulcers, 1.9:1; for asthma,
1.7:1; and for chronic bronchitis, 1.3:1.

the most industrialized regions of the United States, in
New England and the Middle Atlantic States, and is less
prevalent in the South (49-51). Recent figures, however,
indicate that Nevada and California now hold first place
(6.8% and 6.6%, respectively, of the population over 20),
while Hawaii and Alabama are in last place (roughly 1.8% of
the population over 20 (65). In the Soviet Union the
highest level of abstainers is found among Moslems, in the
republics of Central Asia, while the lowest level occurs in
the RSFSR and other Slavic regions. These levels are
identical to those in the United States. An Iowa survey
(66) indicated that 40% of its population were abstainers,
and a California survey (67) found only 13% abstainers. In
the USSR the lower incidence of drinking and especially
alcoholism among Soviet Moslems and Jews can undoubtedly be
attributed to the religious ban against alcohol among the
former and the ritualistic, symbolic meaning of alcohol
among the latter. However, these distinctions are gradually
being erased by the population that is Russian by nationality.
Such nondrinking Russian groups as the Sectarians (Molokans
and others) have now almost disappeared, partly because of
cultural changes and partly as a result of persecutions.

An analogous tendency may be observed in the United
States. Distinct ethnic and religious groups exhibit
different drinking pattern rates (68-82). While a national
American survey revealed no clear cut distinctions in the
drinking patterns of Negro and white men (49-51), other
authors report that alcohol abuse among Negroes, especially
Negro men in urban areas, is several times higher than the
rate for an average cross section of urban society (78-80).
Differences in alcohol consumption among Protestants and
Catholics were also established (69, 71-73, 81). Religious
restrictions play a substantial role among such American
nondrinking cultures as, for example, Baptists, Methodists,
Mormons, and Moslems, although their youth has already begun
to ignore the taboo (50, 51, 72, 75, 76). Although
drinking is widespread among American Jews, the proportion
of heavy drinkers to heavy escape drinkers is lower among
them (50, 51, 70, 72, 74, 77). (This resembles the result
of our survey of the Soviet Union.) It has been shown,
however, that religion in itself is not a decisive factor,
since Irish-American Catholics have different drinking
patterns than Italian Catholics. Bales has pointed out that

the incidence of alcohol problems among Irish-Americans is
consistently two to three times that of other ethnic groups
in the United States (68). At the same time, Italian-
Americans drink more regularly, but they consume their
alcohol during meals and without heavy intoxication (71,
72). Irishmen are comparable to Russian nationals, and
Italians to Georgians and other ethnic groups of the
Caucasus and Moldavia (the "wine" regions).

When American writers discuss cultural differences,
they usually note the ascetic Protestant American view of
alcohol as sinful and point out that the American Jewish
subculture considers drinking as an element that is inter-
twined in the network of sacred ideas; consequently, drinking is learned in a highly controlled, ritualized manner
(70, 72, 76). In contrast to these attitudes, the Irish
male's drinking is seen as dissociated from the network of
religious ideas. The function of drinking is hedonistic
and utilitarian, and drinking is symbolic of hospitality
and sociability (81).* As we mentioned above, the Church
in old Russia exercised little control over drinking
behavior, and the remains of even this weak control have now
vanished. Moreover, drinking has always been a symbol of
enjoyment and hospitality and a tool of social communication
for Russians. It is these elements that explain the
similarity between the Irish and Russian drinking patterns.

It is well known that in America many cultural
distinctions gradually disappear from second- and third-
generation immigrants. The same process is taking place
among young Soviet citizens. This process of the emergence
of an "average" attitude is caused by a number of factors

---

*According to Bales, in Ireland whisky is used "every-
day to begin the day, to get rid of a 'hangover,' to quiet
hunger, to relieve stomach disorders, to get warm, to keep
warm, to reward a child, to release sexual and aggressive
tensions, to relieve emotional difficulties ranging from
minor upsets and disappointments to deep grief, to restore
consciousness in case of fainting and shock, to improve the
physician's skill, to dispel fatigue and to promote sleep--
all of these and more are utilitarian uses, prominently
structured and sanctioned in the Irish culture" (73, p. 185).
There is a similarity between this Irish drinking pattern
and Russian attitudes toward vodka.

in both countries: the weakening of barriers between
cultural patterns, cultural assimilation, integration,
mobility of the population, standardized education, the
mass media, and the decline of old values. The principal
difference between the two countries is found in the type
of drinking norm that is gaining ascendancy. The various
Soviet ethnic groups are adopting the Russian pattern of
"drink to get drunk" and its strong positive attitude toward
drinking. In the United States, on the other hand, more
moderate, general attitudes are prevalent. The heterogeneity
of American society makes it difficult to establish the
influence of a specific national drinking style on the
"average" American pattern. Moreover, the latter shows much
more variation than the "average" Soviet attitude. Both
drinking and abstinence attitudes coexist in many American
communities. In other words, the American cultural attitude
toward drinking is characterized by "social ambivalence,"
which limits the development of stable attitudes such as are
found in certain other cultures (81). As Pittman pointed out
many observers of the American social scene are convinced
that drinking pathologies in that society are perpetuated
by cultural attitudes that veer toward ascetism and hedonism
(81). However, as he noted, drinking gradually becomes an
extreme and uncontrolled form of behavior for many. Skolnick
found many alcoholic complications in groups of students
from abstinent backgrounds (70). According to Skolnick,
individuals who become alienated from their abstinence
backgrounds use excessive drinking as a symbol of revolt
against old values. Even though the ascetic Protestant
traditions of the first immigrants have practically disappeared, "hard" undiluted beverages still are more rarely
consumed in large doses than in Russia. Public drunkenness
with severe intoxication is observed less frequently. In
America all these cases are associated with alcoholism,
while in Russia this kind of drinking behavior is characteristic for a great number of social drinkers.

Let us pass on to the social aspects. While it is true
that the data from the American survey did not confirm the
widely held opinion that the lower class drinks more
frequently than the middle and upper classes, it did reveal
that the former drink to excess more often (49-51). This
is the chief reason for the higher rate of drinking problem
among these social groups. The American upper-upper class
has a permissive attitude toward drunkenness. Dollard (83)

noted that in the upper classes drinking is not a moral
issue but aggressive behavior is penalized. The "cocktail
hour" is an indispensable part of social conduct and contacts for the lower-upper classes. The American upper-
middle class has a neutral attitude toward drinking, while
the lower-middle class reacts negatively to considerable
intoxication. There is much more drinking in the upper-lower
class. Individuals from the lower class usually become
openly aggressive when drinking, particularly toward their
wives and children. Drinking is socially unrestricted in
the lower-lower class (the Saturday-night-to-Monday-morning
bouts). However, contemporary writers assume that Dollard's
observations were to some extent inaccurate. According to
Pittman (81), the cosmopolitanism of the new middle class
in American society today supports the norms of permissive
drinking. For this class, drinking is the path of
emancipation from traditional American values. Lawrence and
Maxwell found that their study can be compared in a very
limited way with Dollard's concept, especially as regards
the upper-middle and upper class levels (84). Stone
correctly notes that status is connected to drinking styles.
At present, drinking style is considered in terms of complex
and shifting status arrangements (85).

I have already discussed the general similarity between
Irish and Russian attitudes toward drinking. The important
differences in these attitudes depend on social factors.
According to our survey, overt "heavy" drinking with
aggressive behavior is more strictly limited among Soviet
party bureaucrats, the military, police, secret service,
and diplomats. Whereas the average Soviet citizen is
open to severe penalties and imprisonment for aggressive
behavior, a member of the Soviet upper class, i.e., the
high Party bureaucracy, is subject only to "moral"
reprimands in the form of a personal chat with his super-
visor or Party colleagues.

Changing attitudes toward drinking and increasing drunkenness among the Soviet middle class may be seen, just as
in the U.S.A., as a rejection of old values, but this is
not the only cause (see below). Drinking behavior in
Russian urban working districts and in so-called urban-type
settlements bears a strong similarity to drinking behavior
in black ghettos in the U.S.A. In neither case is
excessive drinking to the point of heavy intoxication

viewed as deviant. People begin to drink on Friday and
stop on Sunday (some of them are hung over on Monday). The
frequency of alcohol abuse is determined only to a certain
degree by the occurrence of payday. Excessive drinking on
weekends is not considered a sign of alcoholism among
Russian urban male blue-collar workers. In Russia, an
individual is labeled an "alcoholic" only when his behavior
in the intoxicated state becomes excessively aggressive,
when he spends a significant portion of the family budget
on alcoholic beverages, when his social functioning is
disrupted as a consequence of addiction, and when he
successively loses one job after another. Bourne notes
that drunkenness among blacks may be a daily phenomenon.
(They) "can continue for years, and sometimes indefinitely,
to consume small amounts of alcohol all day long without
its interfering with their performance and without significantly decreasing their output. Such a drinking pattern
in a white, middle-class executive would immediately earn
him the label of alcoholic. Whereas in the poor black urban
community it may be viewed appropriately as essential
adaptive behavior" (80, P. 217). This same style of
drinking can be observed in Russia among artisans,
mechanics, plumbers, and other persons who have supplementary sources of income in excess of their primary earnings
(for example, among the numerous speculators and underground
"businessmen"). But an analogous type of drinking behavior,
with regular and occasionally even grave, excesses is also
not infrequent among Soviet writers, artists, actors, and
the "gilded youth." Here, too, alcoholic excesses earn only
a formal, not sincere, condemnation. Moreover, they are
considered a token of bon ton and are even imitated by
neophytes. This, incidentally, is also an old Russian
tradition. Many famous Russian poets, writers and composers
(for example, Blok, Esenin, Kuprin, Musorgskii) abused
alcohol.

Let us review the facts we have presented in this
chapter. As we know, the three original functions of
alcohol have virtually disappeared in contemporary
societies: its religious and medical significance and its
nutritional value (although the latter two functions have
still retained a certain role, especially in Russia). The
rise in drinking in the 20th century has many causes. The
most important among them is the disappearance of taboos
imposed by society, the family, and rituals that limit the

consumption of alcoholic beverages. It is well known that
the expression and extent of these restrictions have varied
greatly from epoch to epoch and in various societies and
cultures, from total abstinence to almost complete permissiveness. The most common sociocultural factors having a
decisive influence on the weakening of this barrier in
modern societies have been, of course, industrialization
and urbanization. These two processes have led to the
disruption and disappearance of restrictions imposed by
culture on the impulse toward gratification, to the degen-
eration of the religious-ritualistic meaning of alcohol,
and to the weakening of the controlling and protective role
of the family. At the same time, social upheavals in the
modern world strengthen feelings of alienation, tension,
anxiety, and escapist reactions, all of which find one form
of expression in drunkenness (86-88). Escapist reactions
increase when an individual cannot satisfy his yearning for
happiness and a meaningful existence through socially and
morally approved forms of activity. Thus, alcohol becomes
the universal solution to problems.

    This is primarily relevant for those groups of the
population that have lost social control, that feel
particularly strongly the downfall of traditional ethical
values, or that express the greatest dissatisfaction with
the status quo. Primary among these are the lower classes,
those who are less well paid, are less educated, and are
discriminated against, as well as young people and women
who demand equal rights and opportunities. According to
Bourne (80), alcohol offers impoverished people an
accessible and immediate pleasure that there is almost no
valid reason to defer. In analyzing these facts, we must
first of all keep in mind that both Negroes and Russian
peasants (whose descendents make up the majority of the
urban communities today) have until fairly recently been
slaves (serfdom was abolished in Russia only in 1861).
According to Engels, drunkenness is a form of protest
against social exploitation, poverty, and the impossibility
of satisfying one's cultural needs. However, the Marxist
interpretation of heavy drinking among underprivileged
groups, as the result of their deprivation and oppression,
is not sufficiently convincing. In fact, during the past
several decades the position of these lower classes has
significantly improved in Russia and especially in America.
The average income of the Soviet blue-collar worker is not

less than that of the white-collar worker or physician
(although all of these earn much less than their American
counterparts). Despite this, however, drunkenness continues
to increase. The Soviet press emphasizes that the basic
cause for drunkenness among "certain groups of the Soviet
population" is not to be sought in economic factors but in
the "absence of cultural interests" (11-13, 16, 18). But
even this is not the main reason. It would be more correct
to speak about the role of the gap between growing expectations and the attained standard of living in circumstances
of the weakening of patriarchal morality and a lack of
spiritual interests. The individual can find nothing to
counter the absence of a meaningful life. An individual's
impression that he is the victim of social injustice and of
unfavorable circumstances is weightier than his low income
level. In other words, while it is true that drunkenness
in the American and Soviet societies, regardless of their
different stratifications and social structures, is more
open and grave among the lower and less educated classes,
this general hypothesis calls for greater specification.
The critics of Dollard's concept have refined this hypothesis
and recognized the fact that membership in a certain class
does not per se explain drinking behavior; it is determined,
rather, by a complex of causes, among which social status,
style of use of the referent group, and the nature of social
control occupy important positions. Thus, as we stated
above, in Russia drunkenness is regular and acute among
certain groups of the intelligentsia and bohemians (among
American bohemians drug abuse is also joined to this), among
Russian artisans, and some other social groups which cannot
be included in the lower and "dissatisfied" classes.

C. The Relation of Drinking to Age and Sex in Both
    Societies

Drinking Among Adolescents

     One of the factors determining the general rise in the
indicators of the use of alcohol in contemporary society is
the inclusion of ever larger segments of young people. We
have already quoted some figures which indicate the high
level of drinking among Soviet and American youth. Public
opinion, taking into consideration the connection between
drunkenness and juvenile delinquency and the moral
deterioration of youth, is expressing concern over this

matter. Despite strict censorship, even the Soviet mass
media are obliged to publish data about drunkenness among
youth with increasing frequency. Thus, for example, an
article, "After the Ball," in the newspaper Sovetskaya
Molodezh (Soviet Youth), describes a typical party in a
so-called "House of Culture" for youth. "Swaying figures
crowded the semi-darkened room. In a corner, a young man
was treating an adolescent to liquor straight from the
bottle. Young girls were trying to ward off the improper
and incoherent advances of drunken youths, but no one
heeded their appeals for help. Broken glass from the entry
door and windows tinkled.... Many staggered around, some
fell down. Entering the foyer, one visitor struck another
in the face.... A fight began." The Soviet newspaper adds
that "such things" occur frequently (89).

The high level of drinking among American adolescents
confirms the theory that in the United States drinking is
learned in adolescence (77, 90). The first drinking
experience tends to occur in the home (91). An analogous
 type of social and cultural learning in adolescence rather
than during childhood, as in France and Italy, predominates
in Soviet society (14). Learning takes place under the
influence of family or friends or both. Thus, the cultural
patterns of the referent group are extremely important.

Youthful alcohol abuse is the manifestation of a
desire to attain adulthood as quickly as possible and
expresses the hedonistic aims of adolescents; for some
modern adolescents it is a form of protest against reality
and an expression of the desire to avoid social responsibility. Both in the United States and in the Soviet Union,
youthful and adolescent behavior was much more strictly
controlled in the past. This could explain the excessive
drinking of youths who have broken away from their fathers'
control (in Russian and Protestant Anglo-Saxon families) or
their mothers' overprotection (in Irish families). At
present, however, the role of the family is growing weaker
both in the Soviet Union and in the United States. Thus,
the spread of drinking among youth can no longer be
attributed to protest. Maddox pointed out that drinking
among teenagers in this society is not primarily a response
to tensions resulting from an anomalous position in social
structure or an expression of hostility toward adult
authority (91). Rather, the opposite is much more likely
to be a causative factor: the role of permissiveness and
overindulgence during childhood, which is a consequence of

the decline of the father-centered family. Some Soviet
authors still speak of the decline of discipline and of
the influence of the family's authority as the cause of
youthful drunkenness. However, there are other important
causes: a youth culture and the identity crisis (92, 93).

In addition, the strengthening of hedonistic tendencies and of the desire to escape the boredom of everday life
play an essential role in youthful drinking. The significance of these factors is well known both in the United
States and in the Soviet Union. Thus, for example, the
Soviet newspaper Komsomolskaya Pravda (Komsomol Truth)
published the following letter written by a 16-year-old
girl: "At our club dances there are both fights and drunk-
en kids, but we've gotten used to it and we like it this
way. What would we do at our dances if we didn't drink?
It would be boring" (94). Girls write to the editor of
another newspaper, Sovetskaya Molodezh: "It's boring at
home, it's boring at the club. What are we to do?" (89).
Drunkenness is the only escape.

Female Drinking

Both countries show an increasing incidence of drinking among women, among whom permissiveness was formerly
less manifest than it is at present. Differences in male
and female alcoholism have been explained, from a sociological point of view, by different role expectations.
These sexual differences, however, are gradually diminishing. The reduction in the ratio of male to female
drinkers and alcoholics is connected not only with the
fact that more women turn to physicians for medical help
but also with the real rise in the number of female
heavy drinkers. The growth of drunkenness among women
is a form of self-affirmation and an imitation of male
customs. The disruption of family ties and female liberation in both societies is an important factor. In
Russia, the consequences of war added to this problem,
with the result that at present there are still 19 million
more women than men. It is true that in the USA the ratio
of female to male heavy drinkers is apparently higher than
in the Soviet Union: respectively about 1:5 (48, 81) and
1:8.5, according to our data (14, 95). According to some
data, the ratio of male to female heavy drinkers is still
higher in the Soviet Union (a group of authors observed

37.1% male heavy drinkers and only 1.9% females among the
employees of a certain institution) (96). These discrepancies between American and Soviet figures apparently do
reflect, in part, the real ratio. In the Soviet Union,
drunkenness among women is still condemned more severely by
society. On the other hand, the Soviet woman fights for
her equality to a lesser extent than the Western woman.
Her chief concern is not female liberation but the preservation of the social and financial stability of the family,
which is threatened by drinking. However, these discrepancies
are also in part explained by the fact that, as a survey of
women in the Soviet Union has shown, Soviet women hide
their alcohol abuses more than do their American counterparts.
Data on the course of female alcoholism are contradictory,
and the problem of comparing the basic clinical symptoms
among male and female alcoholics demands further study. In
the opinion of a number of Soviet authors (14, 25, 36, 46),
female alcoholism has a more acute course and is less
treatable. This is partially due to the fact that the
proportion of underlying emotional disturbances is greater
among women alcoholics than among men.

III. SPECIFIC HISTORICAL, CULTURAL, AND SOCIAL

CAUSES OF DRINKING IN RUSSIA

So far we have focused principally on the analogous
factors that influence the growth of drinking in the Soviet
and American societies. However, there is an entire set of
factors that are exclusive to Soviet society. The first
fundamental difference is connected with historically
determined Russian drinking patterns. We have already
indicated that heavy drinking is typical only for certain
groups within American society. In Russia, however, this
is the comon drinking style. This pattern can be explained
in several ways.

A. The Role of Distilled Spirits and Their Production

It was claimed at one time that Slavic and Northern
peoples, in contrast to Romance groups, have a predilection
for periodic heavy drinking. In this connection,
Montesquieu wrote that this custom is linked to the effect
of the cold climate. These somewhat naive racial and
"geographical" views were subsequently criticized, and at

present differences in drinking style are considered to be
connected with cultural factors and the specifics of
agriculture, which determine the dominant type of alcoholic
beverages in a certain country. For example, drunkenness
with loss of control is related to the predominant use of
distilled spirits. The fact that this form of drinking is
not the exclusive dominion of the Slav race is demonstrated
by the growing consumption of distilled spirits in France.
There are five times as many alcoholics in France as in
Italy. The reason for this is obviously not the fact that
the French drink twice as much as Italians but the fact
that the French consume four times as much distilled spirits
(48, 97). These differences are also related to the fact
that Italians have a much more negative attitude toward
coarse drunkenness. Analogous differences may also be
found among Americans and Russians. Most of the Russian
population have predominatly used and continue to use "hard"
beverages. The Soviet Union has the highest rate of
distilled-spirit consumption in the world. This rate is
twice that of the United States and France. At the same
time, grape wines and light cocktails are used relatively
rarely in Russia. We have already noted that the trend
toward distilled spirits has been increasing in regions
that have traditionally used grape wines. Thus, in Soviet
Georgia, for example, drunken representatives of local
ethnic groups may be seen more and more frequently, while
this used to be more strictly censured. As a result, the
number of alcoholics in Georgia has increased. In addition,
the increase in domestic distillation of alcohol has also
influenced the drinking pattern. Home-brewed liquors are
usually much stronger than wines, have a number of harmful
by-products, and produce more severe intoxication than wines
or commercially distilled spirits. Home-brewing, which
began on a large scale after the passage of the Dry Law at
the beginning of World War I, has at present become widespread not only in the country but also in small cities,
both in Slavic and certain other regions. The cost of
manufactured liquors is the cause for this phenomenon. In
the opinion of the Soviet economist we have already quoted
(8), illegal production of "moonshine" amounts to 50% of
the state production of vodka. We must also take into
account the fact that at one time in the Soviet Union
distilled spirits obtained through special reprocessing of
industrial spirits, from wood or other organic products,
were rather widely used for sale in rural areas. (At present, this practice has allegedly stopped as a consequence of
the increasing number of cases of intoxication).

The Soviet alcohol policy, which we discussed in the
first section, furthers the increasing use of distilled
spirits and consequently the growth of heavy drinking.
Inasmuch as sales of alcoholic beverages, especially vodka,
are fiscally very important for the government, the state
has steadily increased the production of distilled spirits.

B. The Influence of Historical Experience

Among the ancient Slavs, mead and beer were symbols of
both rain, which nourished the earth, and blood. The
ancient Slavic tribes had a tendency toward periodic abuse
of alcohol that was connected with such special events as
funerals, weddings, hunting, harvest, and holidays. The
Scandinavian knights (the Varangians or Normans), who came
to power in Kievan Rus' in the 9th-10th centuries, also
drank a great deal from time to time. In the old chronicles
and byliny (ballads) there are descriptions of magnificent
feasts of princes and their entourages. A large drinking
capacity was considered a feature of a man's strength and
courage. However, the consumption of alcoholic beverages
at this time was predominately a matter of cult and ritual.
Drinking habits of the Eastern Slavs in this period
differed very little from drinking habits among the
Western Slavs and Germanic tribes. People drank in public
drinking-houses (korchmas or taverns) where they also ate,
listened to singers, and discussed community affairs (1).

As a result of the Tatar-Mongolian conquest the South
Russian cities were destroyed. A severe consequence of
200 years under the Tatar yoke was the broken ties with
Western Europe and the decline of economic and cultural
conditions in Russia. The Muscovite state, which arose
in the 15-16th centuries, remained backward in comparison
with Europe. The Tataro-Mongolian khans banned the sale
of alcoholic beverages. The Muscovite grand dukes in
the main followed these restrictions. However, later on,
especially from the time of Ivan the Terrible, the
government, continuing to fight against free public drinking-
houses began to open their own establishments (the so-called
kabaks, which were very profitable for the government). In
contrast to the korchmas, in these establishments it
was possible only to drink, and moreover instead of the

softer mead and beer, they began to sell vodka (1).
Foreigners who visited Moscow in the 17th century noted
the terrible drunkenness in the city. Intoxicated persons,
who not only had spent all their money on drink but also
had sold all their belongings to buy drinks, congregated
around the kabaks.

Thus we can consider that the period after the
liberation from the Tatar yoke was also the period of the
establishment of typical Russian drinking patterns. In
summation, we can describe the following historical and
cultural causes of this: first, the crisis which arose as
a result of the Mongolian conquest, the destruction of the
old cultural patterns and values, and the migration of the
population to northern regions with severer climate; second,
the backwardness of the Muscovite state in comparison with
European states, where attitudes towards drinking gradually
had become more moderate; third, the extended ban on the
sale of alcoholic beverages, and the consequent opening of
the government kabaks, in which the main drink was not mead
and beer, but vodka.

These attitudes toward alcohol abuse in Russian
society changed very little during the 18th and 19th
centuries.

C. The Role of Ethnic Characteristics

The psychological consequences of the above described
historical processes were also fundamental. As I
already noted, the goal of Russian drinking is not euphoria
but heavy intoxication with aggressive behavior. One of
the important national characteristics that predisposes
Russians to such a drinking behavior is the absence of a
sense of proportion and internal discipline, the lack of
restraint and the "passion" of the Russian. The Russian
philosopher Lossky (98) claims that all of Russian history
manifests this passion, this extremism and maximalism. As
evidence for his claim he discusses the Old Believer movement (when hundreds of people immolated or buried themselves
in the name of religion), the fanaticism, martyrdom,
maximalism, and radicalism of Russian revolutionaries, etc.
Even now we witness this martyrdom, this limitless daring
and refusal to compromise, which are incomprehensible to the
restrained and cautious people of the West. (It is sufficient to recall Solzhenitsyn, Sakharov, Bukovsky,

Grigorenko, Marchenko, Plyushch, Kovalev, and many other
Soviet dissidents who have risked their lives for their
ideas.) This trait has been described very well by the
Russian poet A. K. Tolstoy:

> If you love, then love without reasoning,
> If you threaten, then mean it,
> If you swear, then swear rashly,
> If you hack, hack from the shoulder!
> If you quarrel, do it boldly,
> If you punish, punish completely,
> If you forgive, forgive with all your soul,
> If you feast, do it grandly!   (98).

It is also contained in the old Russian proverb, "Drink and
carouse, you live but once!"

As paradoxical as this may be, however, this trait is
juxtaposed with fatalism, passivity, patience, submissiveness,
and laziness. Another Russian poet (and a Slavophile, to
boot), Khomyakov, condemned Russia in these wrathful words:

> Blackened in courts with falsehood black,
> And branded with slavery's yoke,
> With flattery godless, and putrid lies packed,
> You're filled with an infamous, deadening
> Sloth and every vile abomination (98).

Lossky stresses that such an internal contradiction is in
general part of the Russian national character. It is the
cause of such radically differing assessments of Russians
as were made by various foreign visitors and observers, who
sometimes went into raptures over the Russian people and
sometimes described them in the darkest colors.

Another famous Russian thinker, Berdyayev (99) noted
that two contradictory principles lie at the basis of the
Russian soul: the indigenous pagan "dyonisian" and the
ascetic--Christian, Orthodox. This is the source of the
contradictory traits of the Russian people: goodness,
humanitarianism and cruelty, individualism and impersonal
collectivism, universalism and national narrow-mindedness,
the search for God and atheism, meekness and boorishness,
slavery and rebellion. It was not an accident that
Dostoevsky said: "Russian man is broad, it wouldn't be bad

if he became narrower." It is difficult to know the
Russian through and through, and his behavior is always to
a certain degree unpredictable. He is capable of the
noblest and the lowest actions. This is the source of the
polar vacillations of the Russian drunkard's moods; he can
easily pass from infinite love to equally infinite hatred.
He does not admit a middle path. This is the source of
that sharp contrast between his sober and his intoxicated
behavior. When he is drunk he says inappropriate things
(note the Russian proverb, "What the sober man keeps in his
mind, the drunkard has on his tongue") and does things that
are totally opposite to his self-image. In the words of the
Russian historian Pokrovsky, capricious climatic conditions
and economic difficulties have produced in the peasant the
habit of wavering and maneuvering, which conveys the
impression of insincerity and secretiveness. Life has taught
him to live for the moment rather than to anticipate the
future. Lack of self-confidence awakens his powers, while
success shatters them (100).

The spirit of Russian collectivism has found its
expression in the desire to drink in company and to force
alcohol on others.

Many prominent Russian writers and philosophers
(Tolstoy, Dostoevsky, K. Leont'yev, Rozanov, Lossky) have
stressed the anti-individualism, altruism, and deep
religiosity of the simple folk. At the same time, however,
Christian moral values and faith in God instantly vanished
from the consciousness of the Russian during the Revolution
(in the words of Rozanov, they vanished "as though washed
away by water"). Critical periods have brought out such
negative traits of the Russian character as immaturity
(infantility), impulsiveness, a tendency toward elemental
outbursts of cruelty, the herd instinct, and submission to
leaders. Once the Russian begins to doubt an ideal, he is
capable of extreme bestiality and indifference (98).

The great Russian writers and moralists Lev Tolstoy and
Fedor Dostoevsky have depicted in the characters of Platon
Karatayev and Marey a number of traits which they consider
typical of the Russian peasant: goodness, compassion,
wisdom based not on book learning but on a deep love for
man, patience, modesty, moral purity, and trust. Such
people really existed in the Russian village. There is,

however, a striking contradiction between these descriptions and the observations of a number of other Russian realist writers. Thus, for example, Chekhov's story "Novaya Dacha" ("The New Summer House") tells the tale of an engineer and his family who have bought a former gentry estate. These intellectuals loved the folk and tried to establish amicable relations with the peasants. The peasants, however, refused to understand their good intentions and, as the engineer at one point says, "returned evil for good." They chopped down the woods adjoining the estate, stole, were rude, and saw dirty tricks in every attempt that was made to better their lives (101). In the novella "Muzhiki" ("Peasants"), Chekhov described the coarseness, drunkenness, senseless lives, and ignorance of the peasants (102). Another brilliant Russian writer, Bunin, speaks through the hero of his story "Derevnya" ("The Village"): "Is there anything fiercer than our people? In town an entire mob chases a young thief who's grabbed a penny cake off a hawker's tray, and when it catches him forces soap down his throat. Everyone rushes to fires, to fights and is sorry when they end quickly! ...and how delighted they are when someone is beating his wife to death or unmercifully beating a child or amusing himself with him! They teach the mentally retarded to masturbate for pleasure. ...They smear tar on the doors of poor brides (to humiliate them--BMS)! They chase beggars with dogs! They knock pigeons off roofs with stones for amusement! But, you see, it's considered a grave sin to eat these very same pigeons!" Another character in this story exclaims: "You read our history and your hair stands on end: brother against brother, son against father, perfidy and murder (103)".

When the young, idealistic intellectuals "went among the people" at the end of the last century, influenced by the ideas of populism ("Narodniki"), trying to improve the peasant's life, they met with dumb incomprehension, alienation, and even hostility. Thus, for example, in the semiautobiographical novella "Bez dorogi" ("Without a Road"), the writer and physician Veresayev relates the fate of a young doctor who unselfishly tries to treat patients during an epidemic of cholera and is murdered by a drunk, frenzied mob (104).

We have been speaking basically about the peasant-- that "backbone" of the Russian nation. The Russian

intelligentsia was cut off from the people. Although it
did possess a number of typically Russian shortcomings, it
also had unique virtues which made it the conscience of the
nation. Its sense of responsibility and duty to the
people must be especially emphasized. These attitudes of
the Russian pre-revolutionary intellectual elite were shared
by the majority of Russian writers, artists, actors, and
musicians. At the same time, escapist tendencies--the
desire to "escape" prosaic life not only in spiritual spheres
but also in sex and drunkenness-were widespread among them.
The best representatives of the Russian intelligentsia were
brilliantly educated people who held spiritual and intellectual values in the highest esteem.

The smaller cities had a stratum of intelligent,
industrious, conservative, and religious people. Many
Russian "merchants" came from this stratum. On the other
hand, there existed so-called "Meshchanstvo" (petty
bourgeois, philistines), a specific class which had lost
peasant traditions without having acquired true culture.
The narrowness, stupidity, self-satisfaction, and "bestial
customs" of all these people were also often described in
Russian literature. Similar to them was the tremendous
mass of urban clerks and employees, who lacked all spiritual
interests and were devoted only to gluttony and drunkenness.
(See the stories of Gogol', Saltykov-Shchedrin, Chekhov,
Gorky, Kuprin, and other Russian writers.)

In order to understand the causes of the latter
phenomenon, it is necessary to take into account the
following. In psychoanalytical terms it is possible to
speak of the presence of ambivalent attitudes among
Russians, especially with respect to the authorities. The
conjunction of passive-masochistic tendencies with anarchic
impulses gives rise to an internal conflict, which in
particular is manifested in the unrestrained Russian drunkenness, frequently with savage, senseless, and sometimes
even self-destructive cruelty. (An excellent description of
this type of Russian drinking behavior was given by Ivan
Bunin in the story "Ya vse molchu" ("I Keep Silent") (105)).
In severe drunkenness, suppressed aggressive and destructive
impulses are first liberated, and the pressure of the
superego is eliminated; then a sopor develops which imitates
death (escape from life). A general association between thi
type of severe drunkenness and the drive toward self-injury
suggests itself (106). Another important purpose of alcohol

is to free inhibited sexual instincts. As we noted above,
in Russia the consumption of alcohol is a usual way of
establishing sexual contacts and eliminating sexual anxiety.
A drink is a <u>conditio</u> <u>sine</u> <u>qua</u> <u>non</u> of meetings between men
and women which culminate in sexual union. (I was told by a
middle-aged, nonalcoholic worker that "without a drink, it's
somehow embarrassing.") Berdyayev claims that there is
something effeminate in the Russian character, and Lossky
feels that it represents a combination of opposing male and
female positions. It is well known that it is typical for
alcoholics to drink in "male company" and avoid the society
of women (107, 108). It is interesting that in Russia this
tendency is observed not only among alcoholics but among
social drinkers as well. The drinkers usually loudly pro-
claim their disdain for women and stress their traditional
male values--power, and bravery--and simultaneously recount
their successes with women, their sexual abilities, etc.
(This, however, far from always corresponds to reality.)
Thus, totally contradictory characteristics hide beneath
the facade of independence and masculinity. Drunkenness is
also a means of overcoming yet another Russian national
trait: introvertiveness and the closely associated
inability to freely establish social contacts.

All these characteristics are directly tied to the
alcoholic personality (72, 87, 107-115). It is true that
these characteristics may be found in any society, but their
proportion is higher among Russians than among Westerners.
This is the essential cause of the extensive prevalence of
heavy drinking in Russia.

Of course, we have described only a certain "average"
type of Russian, the typical descendent of the Russian
peasantry. In reality there are many exceptions to this.
We must also explain that we do not have in mind genetically
conditioned "racial" traits but the influence of historical
and cultural factors: the lengthy period of the Tatar Yoke,
the three-hundred-year rule of the monarchic-aristocratic
regime, the tardy liquidation of the feudal order of serfdom,
isolation from the general European development, the
relatively late consolidation of the Russian nation (until
relatively recently, the Russian peasant gave his nationality not as "Russian" but as a resident in a specific
province; i.e., "Tambovian" or "Penzian," etc.), the low
cultural level of the people, and the lack of experience

of civic and political freedoms. After a brief period of
democracy (from February to October 1917), the Revolution
culminated in the establishment of a new and even more
repressive, totalitarian form of government. During the
years of Soviet rule the national traits described above
not only were not smoothed over but were intensified as a
result of prolonged social stress.

D. The Social Psychology of Soviet Man as a Factor
    Influencing the Growth of Drinking

      In Soviet society, the individual perceives himself as
totally dependent on the state. His feelings of impotence
and helplessness with respect to the government are much
more strongly expressed than in a pluralistic society. The
experience of long-term political repressions and economic
privation has strengthened the traditional Russian
ambivalence toward power. Worship of strength and power is
one of the reasons for the success of the cult of Stalin,
who filled the vacuum in the soul of the Russian man after
God and "Father Tsar" were debunked. It was not accidental
that the death of Stalin triggered the unfeigned sorrow
of millions of simple people, among whom were many who had
been his victims. Soviet reality teaches man that daring,
aggressiveness, independence, and initiative are punished
and are constantly stifled. Soviet man grows accustomed
to passivity and conformity. From his earliest years, he
is told that the main goal of the ruling Party is concern
for him and his interests. He is used to the thought that
the "authorities" think and decide for him. This breeds in
him a powerful paternalistic orientation. On the other hand,
he daily feels that in reality the bureaucratic machine works
not for him but against him. He cannot obtain his rights
and his desires for the "beautiful life." His salary is far
below the average salary of Western man. His needs are
frustrated. He cannot purchase a color television; his own
home or an automobile are unattainable luxuries for the
overwhelming majority of the population. The services at his
disposal are of very low quality. The average urban man
experiences constant difficulties in purchasing food and
clothing. Even those items that can be found in stores are
of poor quality and assortment. Stores, restaurants, and
service shops all have long lines. The ultimate dream of
Soviet man is to obtain imported clothing (suits, dresses,
shoes, ties) and imported consumer goods (radios, cameras,
etc.). All this can be obtained only with the greatest

difficulty, often only on the black market. People who live
in small towns and in rural areas are in the worst position;
here goods are in even shorter supply than in the major
cities. Although the construction of housing units has significantly accelerated in recent years, there are still not
enough of them. The size of apartments is strictly limited,
and millions of people still live in "communal apartments"
(several families in a single apartment) and wait years for
their turn to receive rooms. At the same time, the Soviet
citizen cannot fail to see that the elite of Soviet society,
which dubs itself the "servant of the people," has barri-
caded itself behind high fences and enjoys all the blessings
of the sweet life at opulent summer homes (see, for example,
H. Smith's description of the life of the Soviet elite)
(116). All this breeds in Soviet man a feeling of dissatisfaction, envy, hostility, anger, alienation, cynicism,
escapism. As a result of the bureaucratization of Soviet
society, the average citizen cannot fulfill his growing
needs and succeed in his desire for success and material
prosperity through legal pathways. It is possible to become
"wealthy," to obtain an apartment out of turn, to purchase
"foreign" goods, to enroll one's children in a privileged
school or university only by breaking the laws, through
speculation, bribery, and foul play. As a result there is
almost no one who does not break Soviet laws, regardless of
the strict persecution and punishment which is meted out to
the "plunderers of socialist property," the bribe-takers,
swindlers, etc. All this produces a rise in feelings of
anxiety and insecurity. The escape from all this is alcohol.

We have been speaking of the Soviet man "in general."
Let us dwell briefly on the sociopsychological preconditions
for drunkenness in various social strata of Soviet society.

Let us begin with the peasantry, that fundamental
bearer of the spirit of "collectivism" in the past. As we
have noted above, the peasantry is vanishing in Russia.
Along with it, as the contemporary dissident philosopher
G. Pomerants notes, the concept of "the people" is
vanishing; only traces of it remain, like little islands
of snow deep in the forest at spring. As a result of this
process, those noble representatives of the people who so
enthralled Tolstoy and Dostoevsky have become a rarity.
(see, for example, Solzhenitsyn's "One Day in the Life of
Ivan Denisovich" and "Matrena's Farmstead.") The shape of

the Russian countryside has changed as a result of
collectivization, the death of the most valuable, "strong"
and sober peasants (the kulaks), and the migration of
healthy young males to the cities. Its patriarchal moral
foundations were rapidly destroyed. The dominant influence
in its sphere has been assumed by the stratum of irresponsible and lazy drunkards, who were relatively few before
the Revolution. This process was even more accelerated by
World War II, when only women, children, and old men
remained in rural areas. The contemporary farmer takes
little interest in working on land that does not belong to
him   Thus, although this farmer is not formally urbanized,
he is in fact alienated from his work. The results of this
were long ago foretold by the Russian writer Gleb Uspensky:
"Tear the peasant from the soil," he wrote, "and a spiritual
emptiness will set in--drunkenness, debauchery, and
swindling" (98).

These processes had an even greater effect on the urban
population, most of whom are of peasant origin. The
consequences of famine, privation, fear, and insecurity
produced by the terror and the destruction of millions of
human lives have been decisively reflected in the psychology
of the typical representative of the contemporary urban
population. In the first years after the Revolution, the
writer Mikhail Bulgakov hinted at the "victory of the proletariat" in his scathing satire "The Heart of a Dog," in
which he depicted the transformation of a dog into a man as
a consequence of an experiment. The result was a sort of
monster lacking both canine and human virtues: a cunning,
cowardly, low, greedy, and dishonorable creature (117).
Mikhail Zoshchenko created a veritable gallery of
representatives of the "new, most perfect contemporary
society." Zoshchenko's Soviet citizen speaks a miserable,
impoverished language, miles away from the beauty of
peasant speech and the diction of cultured people. His
interests are confined to concern about food. He is almost
a beggar, and his expectations are very low. His dreams
revolve around the purchase of new boots or a bottle of
vodka. He has no spiritual interests and he is afraid of
everything. He also knows nothing of love: relations
between men and women are either primitive, mechanical sex,
or searches for pitiful advantage (because in a society of
poverty a "marriage of convenience" gives nothing) (118).

The "amorphous urbanized mass" (119), which grew
tremendously after the Revolution, is very weakly
differentiated both socially and spiritually. There are no
firm boundaries, as had existed before, between workers and
employees. A significant segment of the Party and non-
Party "new Soviet intelligensia" is also spiritually close
to this mass, sharing its system of values and common
origin. This amorphous mass has adopted that spirit of the
petty bourgeoisie, which Russian pre-revolutionary writers,
intellectuals, liberals, and revolutionaries so insistently
mocked and hated. These people have totally lost all
vestiges of the peasant sense of duty and faith in God,
without, however, acquiring a new morality. For them,
Communist ideals are an empty sound, and higher spiritual
values do not exist at all. But as Goethe noted, the
religion of duty may only be replaced by higher values. If
this does not happen, then a "bare man" arises on the "bare
earth," in the words of the Russian writer L. Andreyev.

The new urban generation has received a formal education
and a taste for the external attributes of the "cultured
life" (fashionable dress, the cinema, etc.), but it has not
developed true spiritual and esthetic values (Solzhenitsyn
calls this phenomenon "obrazovanshchina"--petty, banal,
superficial education). It has lost its ties with the
countryside, disdains the "village muzhiks" and their
"boorishness" and "stupidity," even though it is morally
inferior to them (see, for example, the contemporary
stories of V. Maksimov, V. Shukshin, and V. Lipatov) (120-
122). D. Merezhkovsky, in describing the threat of the
approach of the petty bourgeoisie, called it the "Future
Ham." Like their pre-revolutionary predecessors, the
Soviet petty bourgeoisie are permeated with an authoritarian spirit, conservative, filled with complexes of envy
and militant egoism, greedy, unprincipled, hypocritical,
chauvinistic, xenophobic, and antisemitic.

The growth of expectations of this powerful stratum of
Soviet society offers a contrast to the description of
Soviet man given by Zoshchenko in the 1920s and 1930s. He
is no longer content with his "daily bread" and pair of
trousers. He has seen foreign films and many of his
compatriots have been in the West, both during the war
and after it. The government, however, is not able to
satisfy these growing expectations.

These sociopsychological factors are the cause for
the growth of drinking among all strata of the urban
population, although the distinctive features of the status
of various segments of this population influence the form
of drinking behavior. As regards the new intelligentsia,
only the most average, unprincipled, and limited careerists
survived and prospered in the conditions of the Stalinist
"artificial selection." Writers, philosophers, historians,
all those who were earlier the conscience of the nation,
were now compelled to glorify and serve the regime. The
most blatant toadies, who produce untalented but profitable
books, paintings, and operas, have successful careers, receive prizes, travel abroad. The contemporary dissident
poet A. Galich has created a series of portraits of these
semi-petty bourgeoisie, these semi-intellectuals, time-
servers, careerists, whose motto is to keep silent, curry
favor with the authorities, disdain the weak, and betray
friends. Their aim in life is tasty food, plenty of liquor,
and a secure life.

Only a part of the intellectuals can be termed
spiritual descendants of the Russian intelligentsia. These
nonconformists and dissidents champion the spiritual values
of Russian culture and courageously campaign for freedom
and democracy. However, the general situation of
spiritual crisis, the necessity for constant lying and
concealing of one's thoughts or of expressing them under
threat of persecution, even among this part of the intelligentsia breeds escapism, and particularly a rise in
drinking. Thus, drunkenness is the universal means of
those who have primitively hedonistic aims as well as of
those who are pressured to renounce their spiritual and
esthetic values.

Our discussion paints a rather somber picture of
human degradation that recalls F. Nietzche's depiction of
the "last man," who "makes everything small," or the gloomy
fantasies of G. Orwell. But is all this the distinctive
feature of Soviet man? And here we must answer, "no."
Everything the intellectual critics have said about Soviet
man is just. But in essence we are talking about universal
human vices and the problems of contemporary civilization.
Social systems do not form a new type of "homo sapiens."
At various stages of the development of society, more
altruistic human tendencies alternate with more antisocial
ones. Thanks to the mechanisms of learning, a culture can

favor some qualities and impede others. We have already
noted that the Soviet petty bourgeoisie differs little from
its pre-revolutionary counterpart. (Mayakovsky has already
said that "when the Revolution had thundered by, the mug
of the petty bourgeois peered behind the back of the RSFSR.")
Moreover, as we already remarked, thanks to analogous, though
slower, processes of urbanization and the destruction of
patriarchal and Judeo-Christian values, the West has also
been producing a growing stratum of "the urbanized mass,"
bereft of the old values and striving only for material,
and not spiritual, culture. This, in part, explains the
growth of crime and drinking. If we are to approach
Western man with the same high standards by which some
Russian (and sometimes Western) moralists, philosophers,
and writers measured him, then we can find in him also a
mass of negative traits: egoism, loss of spiritual
interests, amorality, hypocrisy, chase for success and
material values, greed, national prejudices, faith in
authority, conformity, and other well known human qualities.

Despite all this, Soviet man possesses a number of
psychological traits, generated on the one hand by historical
and cultural patterns and on the other by social experience
that was more difficult than in the West. In sum, he is to
a greater degree characterized by anxiety, hostility, envy,
dissatisfaction, and ambivalence toward power. The result
of this is escape into drinking.

E. Some Theoretical Inferences on the Causes of Drinking
    in Russia

Thus, Soviet society, in addition to a number of
factors favoring drinking that are common to all
industrialized societies, has a number of specifically
unique motives. In particular, the possibilities for
self-realization and for expression of one's creative
initiatives are frustrated in a closed society. Drinking
becomes one of the few permissible paths to the
realization of suppressed activity. Moreover, a vacuum
has developed in the spiritual life of the people, since,
on the one hand, they have been deprived of traditional
faith and ethical values and, on the other, they have
become disillusioned with the Communist ideology. According
to Horton, drinking tends to be accompanied by a release of
sexual and aggressive impulses and the strength of the
drinking response in any society tends to vary directly with

the level of anxiety in that society (123). But this
hypothesis is not altogether correct even with respect to
primitive societies (124). True, some social processes
have brought about a situation in which in contemporary
closed societies the role of anxiety has grown, making
them similar to primitive societies. Moreover, in discussing a theory of motives, we must consider more than the
desire to reduce anxiety and to compensate for and minimize
some other psychological problems, as well as to escape
from social stress. Based on the law of causality, the
concept of drinking behavior is also needed in other
modifications. This "law" reflects only a partial norma-
tiveness. Individuals and societies not only reveal the
desire to reduce tension and avoid unpleasantness but also
use the antihomeostatic model of behavior. The essence of
the latter consists of the creation of tension where it does
not already exist (125). This may be called "escape from
boredom." It is important not only that Russian children
taste alcohol rather early but also that the child grows
up in circumstances where regular and heavy drinking is the
rule.

Thus, the socialization process in Russia includes not
merely learning to use alcohol on ritual days and in
response to stress, as is the case in other societies, but
to abusing alcohol in any situation at all. As we have
already noted, the sociopsychological consequences of
migration and assimilation have led to the present
increasing adoption of the drinking pattern characteristic
for the Russian national majority by a broader and broader
group of young males and females of urban and rural areas
of the Soviet Union. Its spread is favored by traditional
permissiveness toward drinking. Russian drinking customs
are now an almost universal phenomenon, and this puts an
extremely strong psychological pressure on nonconformists
who try to avoid the informal socially prescribed forms
of behavior. Drinking is one of the ways of belonging to
a social group.

IV. A COMPARISON OF METHODS OF RESEARCH,

TREATMENT, AND PREVENTION

A. American and Soviet Approaches to the Study of the
    Etiology of Alcoholism

Above we examined some aspects of the problem of
drinking. As regards the etiology of alcoholism, American
works in this area are considerably more heterogeneous
and numerous than Soviet studies.

Since we cannot examine this question in detail here,
we shall note only the following. It is customary to
distinguish the sociological, physiological, and
psychological theories of alcoholism, although at present
some studies bear a multidisciplinary character. In the
United States there are many sociological hypotheses that
in essence examine the causes of drinking but not the
etiology of alcoholism. Soviet authors, although in
accord with the Marxist-Leninist philosophy emphasizing
the crucial role of social factors in the genesis of
alcoholism, touch on these questions rarely and only
superficially, limiting themselves to stating the influence
of the social group (the "micro-environment").

In experimental research conducted on animals, American
physiologists and biochemists attempted to establish a link
between damage to specific organs or the inadequacies of
specific metabolic products, alimentary factors, enzymes and
vitamins, and craving for alcohol: hypotheses on the role
of disruptions of the metabolism of catecholamines,
hypoadrenocorticism, damage to the liver, deficiencies of
the group B vitamins, hyperactivity of the cholinergic
structures of the brain, etc. (See, for example, Kalant's
review (126)). These studies, however, have more than once
been criticized for their methodology and some of the data
were subsequently not confirmed. Soviet experiments on
animals have essentially been devoted to the toxic effect
of alcohol on the organism. Relatively recently, reports
have appeared on the formation of a "craving" for
alcohol (27).

Some American research demonstrating the role of stress
and anxiety in intensified alcohol consumption in animals

approaches psychological theories (see below); another
important area of research deals with the chemical and
pharmacological features of alcohol, the effect of acute
and chronic intoxication on the cerebrum, liver, endocrine
and metabolic functions; a certain number of works is
devoted to the effects of alcohol on psychological
response (motor, auditory, and visual skills), on perception
and cognition (64, 72, 87, 97, 127-129). These approaches
and hypotheses that are based on them are fully shared by
Soviet scholars. However, very few corresponding Soviet
works have been published in this area, due to insufficient
interest on the part of the major laboratories in the
problem of the etiology of alcoholism. According to
Roebuck and Kessler (86), the next group of psychological
theories may be characterized as having a "reinforcement
orientation." This orientation, based on the conception
of learning and stimulus-response theories, is close to
traditional Soviet works, which are based on the theory of
conditional reflexes. Yet another group of psychological
works is connected with "transactional orientation" and
stresses the role of interpersonal processes and social
roles in the development of alcoholism. The psychoanalytical approach is first of all based on Freud's conception
of the role of latent homosexuality and fixation on oral
eroticism in the development of alcohol abuse, which
returns the alcoholic to his infantile childhood sexual
experiences (108, 109). Here a number of authors stress
the difference between social or "reactive" drinkers, who
use alcohol to separate their "ego" from the external world
and addictive alcoholics, who suffer from "oral perversion"
(72). Other studies with a psychoanalytical orientation
point to the significance of feelings of guilt, inferiority
masochism, depression, hostility, aggression and auto-
aggression, dependency, loneliness (109, 110, 113-115, etc.
Reviewing various psychological theories, Roebuck and
Kessler arrive at the conclusion that "alcoholics are
basically dependent personalities which have turned to
alcohol as a means of escape from internal and external
stress" (87).

Later psychodynamic works call attention to the role
of tension and anxiety and the inadequacy of the individua.
adaptive possibilities. All these writers give special
significance to the person's early experience and to his
relations with his parents. This problem, however, is far
from being so simple. Thus, for example, McCords

reported that two forms of discipline were often found in the alcoholics' families; alcoholics' fathers were varied in their demands: they would punish a certain act and at other times they would ignore the same action. Thus "erratic punitiveness and laxity are significantly involved in the causation of alcoholism and crime" (110). To a certain degree, attempts to isolate specific personality traits predisposing a person to alcoholism are close to this orientation.

As we noted above, Soviet psychiatrists have denied the significance of all studies in this area. They have termed the psychoanalytical interpretation of alcoholism "anti-scientific" and reactionary (3, 25, 37, 46). As regards the study of the alcoholic personality, the Soviet position has to a certain degree loosened in this respect, and at the present time a number of works acknowledge that certain emotional disorders may accelerate the development of alcohol addiction. The theory of the role of disrupted family relations, parental conflict, and the significance of an early experience of alcohol has gained greater acceptance in the Soviet Union. Almost all Soviet studies now emphasize the importance of these factors.

As regards early tasting of alcohol, it was formerly held that addiction in these cases proceeds more rapidly. Later, however, attention was brought to the fact that the first drinking experience among Jews usually occurs very early (often before the age of 7), while alcoholism is an extremely rare phenomenon in this group. Ullman (130) reported that American addictive drinkers had their first drink at a later age than nonaddictive drinkers. According to our data (14), 65% of addictive alcoholics began to use alcoholic beverages before the age of 18, and 80% before the age of 20. However, early use of alcohol did not accelerate the development of the basic symptoms of alcoholism. In groups with early and late (after the age of 20) initiation to drinking, addiction symptoms appeared at the same age. In other words, in cases of later initiation to drinking, addiction symptoms frequently appeared even more rapidly. An exception to this was a group of young alcoholics with a "malignant" process course, in which manifest prealcoholic emotional disorders were observed. It was reported in the United States that "early alcohol problems per se may not explain later alcohol problems, but some unique sets or

combination of early drinking problems may well explain
later serious drinking problems more effectively than
others" (88, IV).

Finally, American and Soviet studies frequently assert
that aging lowers the intensity of alcohol craving.

Let us draw some conclusions from this analysis.
Individual contemporary Soviet works support the conclusion
of a number of American researchers that the development of
heavy drinking is favored by the following factors:
positive attitudes toward drinking and environmental support
of heavy drinking, urbanization, emotional instability,
alienation and maladjustment, unfavorable expectations, and
looseness of social control. Sex, age, and socioeconomic
status influence this process. All this, however, still
does not explain the causes for the development of alcohol
addiction. In American as well as Soviet society there
exists a large group of social drinkers (not neurotics,
psychopaths or psychotics) who become alcoholics only after
15 to 20 years of alcohol abuse. But in any society there
are individuals in whom the addictive process takes a very
rapid course. These are persons with certain emotional
disorders, who move from social drinking to addictive
alcoholism without manifesting any nonaddictive problem
phase. In the Soviet Union this group of "neurotics and
psychopaths" comprises only one-fourth to one-fifth of all
addictive alcoholics, while the figure is apparently
higher in the United States. This supports the hypothesis
that the more widespread excessive drinking is in a given
society, the smaller the proportion of pathological
predisposition among alcoholics. It is also interesting
that American reports usually show a higher incidence of
alcoholism among the parents of alcoholics than do Soviet
ones. Some authors cited figures of 52% (131). According
to my data, however, only 10% of the alcoholic patients'
parents were alcoholics. But in 70% of the cases, the
parents used and abuse alcoholic beverages, while among
friends drinking took place in 93% of all cases (14). Thes
data tend to support the view of the influence of the socia
environment rather than of hereditary factors. According
to Roebuck and Kessler (87) there is evidence of some
hereditary predisposition factors in alcoholism. Some
contemporary Soviet writers would agree with their statement that there is not an hereditary predisposition toward
alcoholism per se but that there are factors of heredity

which predispose an individual to many types of
pathological behavior and that one of these under certain
environmental conditions might be alcoholism (87).

American and Soviet physiological, biochemical, and
genetic studies offer much interesting information on the
effect of alcohol on bodily functions. To date, however,
there are no reliable data that would make it possible to
formulate an adequate and fundamental biochemical
(physiological) theory of the etiology of alcoholics. In
particular, we cannot yet explain the mechanisms of
addiction and the role of genetic factors.

B. A Comparison of Diagnostic Criteria and the Concept
of Disease

In both the United States and the Soviet Union, the
concept of alcoholism as a disease has only relatively
recently received broader recognition; even today a
considerable part of the population continues to view this
problem from a strictly moral perspective. Since we cannot
give a history of the various classifications of alcoholism
and describe the numerous American concepts of it, we will
limit ourselves to noting the following: as a result of
Jellinek's contributions (132) and investigations of the
1950s devoted to the withdrawal syndrome (133, 134), many
contemporary American studies place a strong emphasis on
the crucial role of alcohol addiction and physical
dependency. American writers also use several other
criteria (epidomiological, behavioral, sociological, legal),
while Soviet writers rely essentially on clinical criteria.
This difference can be explained by the fact that in the
Soviet Union problems of alcoholism were until recently
studied exclusively by psychiatrists. Their position with
respect to the diagnosis of "alcoholism" is at present
closer to the position of American psychiatrists than was
the case some 20 to 25 years ago (9, 14, 25, 29-32, 36, 40-
46).

Nonetheless, certain differences remain. In the West,
Jellinek's concept (132), which holds that the course of
alcoholism passes through a number of phases, has become
widespread. A multidisciplinary approach is used in the
analysis of the development of these phases; along with
such criteria as physical dependency, various psychological
reactions of the alcoholic are also taken into account.

Thus, for example, the sense of guilt is explained psycho-
logically. In Soviet concepts of alcoholism as a disease,
the clinical approach prevails (9, 14, 29-32, 40-46), and
particularly the sense of guilt and some other symptoms are
seen as signs of the alcohol abstinence syndrome.

C.   Prevention and Treatment Approaches

One of the most essential differences between the USA
and Russia, relating to prevention, is the fact that the
temperance movement has always had a greater influence in
the USA. In Russia, "sobriety societies" began to be organized only shortly before the Revolution. They never achieved
a significant influence on the people and were liquidated by
the Soviet regime. They have so far not been reintroduced,
despite the fact that this question is discussed in the Soviet press. The second basic difference may be found in the
fact that in the United States the Protestant Church, certain other religious sects, and Judaism have negative attitudes toward drinking. The Russian Orthodox Church, however,
as we noted in the introduction, never held such a severely
condemning position, and after the Revolution, along with the
decline in religious life, the role of religious restrictions
was almost completely eliminated.

The system of contemporary preventive measures in the
USA and in the Soviet Union cannot be called exemplary or
consistent. Government, union management, and several other
programs exist (63, 88, 97, 115, 127, 129, 131, 135-138).
In the USA some preventive work is done by the National
Council on Alcoholism (NCA), the National Institute on
Alcohol Abuse and Alcoholism (NIAAA), Alcoholics Anonymous
(AA), and the clergy. The Soviet Union has corresponding
establishments in the form of groups and councils that are
organized in the campaign against alcoholism in some of the
large factories. However, in both countries the intensity
of this preventive work, as well as the funds expended on
it, do not by far compare with other programs, such as cance
prevention and research. In the past both nations attempted
to enact "dry laws." As we noted above, Soviet attempts to
combat drunkenness by limiting the hours of sale and raising
the price of "hard" liquor, curtailing its production, etc.,
have been unsuccessful. Although the USA, like the Soviet
Union, has laws in some states limiting the sale of alcohol,
especially to minors, they are not always strictly observed.

In the United States, primary prevention, i.e., measures designed to impede excessive drinking, takes the form of educational measures, while in the Soviet Union it is carried out as so-called antialcohol propaganda. These measures, however, rarely reach the young people, to whom they should primarily be addressed. Both countries make inadequate use of systematic education aimed at children and teenagers to promote a negative attitude toward alcohol abuse. The matter is usually confined to teachers' formal comments on the hazardous effects of alcholic beverages.

Soviet and American families are usually equally ineffectual, in part because of declining authority and in part because the parents themselves not infrequently consume alcoholic beverages.

Connor (139), in speaking of Soviet preventive measures, asks, "How many potential heavy drinkers are affected by antialcoholic propaganda? How many are influenced by the attitudes of that portion of the Soviet public, however small it may be, which is really 'antidrink'?" To these questions we may answer: very few. But this pessimistic conclusion apparently may also be extended to the American prevention system. Of course, in both cases we unfortunately do not have precise statistical data, but this conclusion is indirectly supported by the growth of heavy drinking and the drunkenness of the young generations. As in any other area, the problem lies in the fact that explanations and arguments have little effect on attitudes that are usually formed at an early age and depend more on the attitudes of the referent groups than on the opinions of the mass media and officials This conclusion is supported by the numerous discussions of the possibilities of changing social attitudes (see, for example, 140).

In the USA, some typical nonspecific measures that indirectly aid primary prevention of alcoholism among the lower classes are desegregation, the fight against poverty, and measures to improve the education and progress of minority groups.

Unlike the Soviet Union, and in accord with the tradition of the Western world, the United States does not use such measures of secondary prevention as public censuring of a drunkard's behavior at meetings, the "influence of shame," etc.

With respect to the organization of alcoholism treatment, American alcoholics are treated on an outpatient basis in clinics, special centers (especially community mental health centers), psychotherapeutic facilities, social service and Alcoholics Anonymous groups, day and night hospital facilities, and by private practitioners (including psychiatrists); alcoholics with physical or psychic complications are admitted to general or mental hospitals; finally, there are custodial institutions for "burned-out" alcoholics (63, 97, 115, 127, 129, 131, 136, 138). The choice of the place of treatment depends on the individual case and the resources and desires of the patient. The Soviet two-step system of mental health centers (dispensaries) and hospitals that service specific districts is free and doubtlessly more efficient. Therefore, it is more effective than the American system of care for alcoholics. The deficiency of the latter is the lack of planning, accounting, and control and the fact that the quality of care depends on the patient's economic status. Its advantages are its greater flexibility and the existence of social workers, psychologists, and counselling programs that do not exist in the Soviet system of mental health services. Moreover, as we noted above, in the Soviet Union only the major cities offer more or less well organized care and prevention. This is also true for America. Thus, in both societies qualified care is not sufficiently and uniformly available to all groups of the population.

In contrast to the United States, where compulsory treatment is relatively rarely used, the Soviet Union widely exploits this system (33-35). The fact that this system was created reflects not only the general tendencies of the Soviet government but also the greater threat of alcoholism to Soviet society.

The principles of the therapeutic process and indications for outpatient and inpatient treatment are very similar. In both countries, the outpatient method is generally considered preferable for less acute cases and hospitalization for cases with considerable psychic and physical complications (9, 14, 23, 31, 34, 35, 36, 40, 41-46, 97, 115, 127, 129, 131, 136-138).

In the United States the patient's personality has greater significance than in the Soviet Union, where a biological orientation still predominates. For this reason psychotherapy is more broadly applied in the United States. In addition, three techniques for behavioral modification predominate: individual psychotherapy, group psychotherapy, and the group approach used by the AA. Such special techniques as psychodrama, hypnosis, and aversive therapy are rarely applied. Treatment of the families has been found to help in the recovery of alcoholics. In recent years, transcendental meditation has been used more and more extensively; its principles are to a certain degree close to those of the autogenic training used in the Soviet Union (14, 39, 95).

American aims and methods of psychotherapy have traditionally been contrasted to Soviet ones, with the latter being characterized as more authoritarian, didactic, and paternalistic, ignoring the role of the unconscious sphere and of inner conflicts and appealing to the consciousness and to social responsibility. In recent years, however, these differences have been smoothed over to a certain extent. True, suggestion, autogenic training, and so-called "rational therapy"--i.e., persuasion, explanation of the incorrectness of the patient's behavior--are more widely used in the Soviet Union, while group therapy based on discussion is preferred in the United States. However, a certain convergence has taken place in this area. Americans are relying more and more rarely on classical psychoanalysis and more often on eclectic methods, although they do take into account the early emotional experience of the patient and the ego's defense mechanisms. Although Soviet psychotherapists continue to negate the psychoanalytical orientation, they are modifying their position as they gain a greater understanding of the emotional problems of the personality (14, 26, 37, 141-143).

The latest works on psychotherapy published in both countries reveal similar ideas expressed in almost identical terms. The therapist is advised to use an individualized rather than a stereotyped approach to the patient. He should not moralize, preach, lecture, but understand the emotional problems of the patient, show him sympathy, give him support and encouragement, help him accept his illness and free himself from the feeling of dependency, realize

his true problems and overcome the avoidance of difficulties
and frustrations through drinking, develop a feeling of
greater responsibility and a more mature approach toward
decision-making, etc. (14, 37, 97, 115, 197, 131, 136,
141-143). Both American and Soviet specialists state that
group therapy has a number of advantages over individual therapy, since the patient often accepts the criticism and suggestions of other alcoholics more readily than those of the
doctor. Interactions, meetings, and discussions help him
to identify himself as an alcoholic and to free himself
from such defense mechanisms as denial, from feelings of
resentment, fear, anger, depression, guilt, and loneliness.
Both American and Soviet writers indicate that the
therapist should play the most active role in the beginning
of the treatment process in order to maintain an adequate
focus in the discussions and should later increasingly
include the collective factors of interaction. It is
interesting to note that the preference for collective
therapy over individual therapy is in both countries
motivated not so much by the patient's immaturity and lack
of intellectuality as it is with his limited financial
resources.

I doubt whether the paternalistic principles of Soviet
psychotherapy are a serious handicap, since paternalistic
attitudes are typical for the Russian alcoholic. If it
proves to be useful to satisfy this need, there is no
basis for avoiding this mechanism in therapy. The Soviet
therapists' lack of familiarity with contemporary concepts
of the personality in behavioral motives is a much more
basic deficiency. This makes it impossible to deeply
understand the inner feelings of the patient, those feelings
which all Soviet authors insist must be understood.

The therapist's theoretical concepts and chosen
methods, however, do not pose as much of a basic problem as
do such factors as his interest in his work and the amount
of time he can spend on such a demanding patient as an
alcoholic. Psychotherapy in the United States and in the
Soviet Union is in many cases unfortunately limited to
several sessions; far too few of them are devoted to
"behavioral modification," and the doctor has neither the
opportunity nor the time for lengthy observation and
treatment of the patient. Moreover, it is obvious that without after-care alcoholics usually quickly suffer relapses.

The similarity of therapeutic approaches becomes evident to an even greater degree in the area of medical treatment. In both countries virtually the same drugs are used for detoxification, for suppressing the withdrawal syndrome, and for improving the metabolic processes, the patient's mental state, sleep, and appetite. Both American and Soviet authors recommend the cautious prescription of tranquilizers (especially librium and valium and their analogues) and when there is evidence for their necessity, antipsychotic drugs (major tranquilizers); sedatives, anti-depressants and psychic energizers are more rarely prescribed. In all cases, American and Russian physicians give vitamins, adequate nutrition, and hydration to normalize the metabolic processes. Finally, "protective" drugs, mainly disulfiram (antabuse), lycopodium selago, etc., are prescribed. Although antabuse remains one of the favorite methods of treatment, a lowering of its effective-ness has been reported. Thus, while in the 1950s antabuse treatment in the Soviet Union yielded as a rule a one to two year abstinence from alcohol, now such remissions have become exceptional as a result of the fact that the public has been given information on the short-term effect of this drug. Another reason for greater skepticism toward antabuse is the finding that it produces various complications.

There are a few drugs which are prescribed only by Soviet or only by American doctors: dithiol compounds and sodium thiosulfatum in the Soviet Union (14); and several others in the United States.

A number of American works emphasize the value of combining the AA with medical treatment and a multidis-ciplinary therapeutic approach. Fox points out, "I believe that 60% to 80% of the well-motivated middle- and upper-income patients who have attempted such a multidisciplinary type of therapy...and who will pursue it faithfully for one to two years will recover" (130). This is absolutely correct for Soviet society as well, but here the problem lies in supplying all of these conditions.

American and Soviet contemporary studies emphasize the important role of psychotherapy, follow-up treatment and maintaining counselling contact with the staff, and the importance of establishing normal social and family relations. However, contrary to Soviet authors, American psychiatrists

assign crucial significance to the alcoholic's personality
and note that abstinence does not solve his emotional
problems. Such an approach is consistent with the Western
psychiatric tradition which holds that alcoholism is a
symptom of an underlying personality problem, for example,
orally fixated infantile character, etc. In a 1967 survey
only 7% of American psychiatrists said that they tried to
help the patient attain abstinence; more than half of the
psychiatrists tried to modify the underlying emotional
problems (138). This approach is apparently correct, but
in practice it results in the psychiatrist's not demanding
total abstinence, which hinders the success of treatment.
In other words, as Joan Curley rightly notes, "It sounds
reasonable, but it rarely works" (144). The same may be
said of the assertions of Soviet psychiatrists on the
necessity of "restructuring the alcoholic's attitudes,"
socially rehabilitating him, etc. Russian physicians have
neither the time nor the possibilities for realizing these
tasks.

     A comparison of treatment results in both countries
shows that the effectiveness of alcoholism medication
and of psychotherapy depends not so much on the type of
drugs as on the organization of the treatment process and
the quality and duration of after-care. Despite the fact
that alcoholism is recognized as a social and medical
problem, both Soviet and American doctors often work in
isolation from social and educational institutions.

     American writers' evaluations of the effectiveness of
therapy also fluctuate widely. An evaluation of the rate
of "socially recovered" alcoholics, according to various
data, vacillates between 10% and 80%. For example,
according to Wallerstein (137), a total improvement rate is
as follows: antabuse therapy, 53%; conditioned reflex
therapy, 24%; group hypnotherapy, 36%; milieu therapy,
26%. A significant number of the writers do not express
any great optimism and report the average rates of
effectiveness as 24% to 44%. Summing up various data
(9, 14, 23, 34, 35-46, 97, 115, 127, 131, 137,138, and
others), we may say that both in the Soviet Union and in
the United States only about one-third of the cases show a
good effect for periods exceeding a year after discharge.
Thus, it is possible to consider that on the average the
data for both countries are very close and depend on

identical factors. The activity of Alcoholics Anonymous
presents an exception to this. AA reports considerably
longer periods of sobriety for former alcoholics. The same
may be said for those individual Soviet psychiatrists who
use the principles of "re-education" ("Makarenko's method").

Finally, it should be said that neither country gives
enough prestige to the problems of research and management
of alcoholism, not only in medical, but also and particularly in governmental and scientific circles. Changes in
American public attitudes toward alcoholism date only from
the recent past, and a negative image of the alcoholic still
prevails among medical personnel (88). As we already noted,
an analogous situation exists in Soviet society, which to
this day widely holds the opinion that alcoholism is a
problem of a moral nature. Even psychiatrists hold these
negative attitudes: at the same time as American psychiatrists consider alcoholism to be a much less important and
interesting problem than neuroses or psychopharmacology,
Soviet psychiatrists believe that the problem of alcoholism
can in no way be compared with the problem of psychoses,
especially schizophrenia. All this partially explains why
in both countries there are insufficient funds for research
in the field of alcoholism. Despite the sophisticated
equipment of American laboratories and the high quality of
several physiological, biochemical, and pharmacological
studies, a relatively small number of new, effective
methods have been proposed for the treatment of alcoholics
in the United States.

Conclusion

Despite the differences in historical, cultural and
social conditions between the Soviet Union and the United
States, drinking and alcoholism are at the present time a
most serious problem for both societies.

Both the United States and the Soviet Union have
considerable differences in the incidence of drinking and
alcoholism among various social and cultural groups of the
population. Specifically, these figures are highest in
the Soviet Union among blue-collar male workers in the
Slavic and Baltic regions and in the United States among
Irishmen and in black ghettos. Drinking in the middle
class is usually more controlled in both countries. But

the social status and the reference group, rather than
"class" affiliation, exert an especially marked effect on
drinking behavior. At the same time the tendency toward
a gradual lessening of differences conditoned by cultural
background, social and sex factors, especially among
youth, is observed in both societies. In Russia, the
growth of drinking occurred first of all as a result of the
increase in the urban population, the adoption of the
Russian drinking pattern by the Russian peasantry and the
minorities, and the new drunkenness of a significant
number of young men. Although in the Soviet Union the
number of female heavy drinkers has been growing, the
greater conservatism of Russian society has made the
proportion of female to male alcoholics lower than in the
United States. According to the findings of a number of
American and Soviet writers, the incidence of alcoholism
decreases with advancing age.

The data we have cited testify to the fact that
alcoholism in a very real sense threatens the health of the
population and does great damage to the social and
economic lives of both countries. On the basis of such
figures and the rate of consumption of distilled spirits,
however, the Soviet Union has outdistanced the United States
in the incidence of drinking and alcoholism, the number of
violations and crimes connected with intoxication.

It is difficult to assess the results of psychological
studies in both countries, especially of a number of
American publications. We may conclude, however, that in
the Soviet Union and in the United States the personality
variations of the majority of social drinkers fluctuate
within the bounds of the hypothetical norms. At the same
time, American and some Soviet data show that cases from
"broken homes," with maladjustment, dependency, intolerance
to frustrations, anxiety, tendencies to impulsive and
self-punishing types of behavior, sense of guilt, isolation
and hostility, and sexual problems occur proportionately
more frequently among alcoholics than among nonalcoholics.
However, the percentage of underlying emotional disorders
is perhaps smaller among Russian alcoholics than among
American alcoholics.

Of the various social and psychological theories of
drinking, the theory of social learning is apparently the

most productive. Nonetheless, mechanisms of alcohol
addiction call for a physiological and biochemical interpretation.

There are several common social causes for the growth
of drinking in the Soviet and American societies. In the
first place, the influence of urbanization and its
psychological consequences, the weakening of social control
and cultural taboos, the decline of the protective influence
of the family, the adoption of the positive drinking
attitudes of the majority and social learning during
adolescence belong here. The influence of these common
factors primarily affects the young generation as well as
the dissatisfied social strata whose expectations are
greater than real opportunities. These people's conviction
that they are victims of society is an important motive
of drunkenness.

However, there are also a number of differences. The
basic one is conditioned by the traditional Russian drinking
pattern, with its tendency to drink to the point of manifest
intoxication and almost total permissiveness. This type of
drinking behavior is determined by the consumption of
distilled spirits and is linked with early Russian
historical experience and also cultural and psychological
characteristics, particularly such traits as ambivalent,
sado-masochistic attitudes, introvertiveness, lack of
self-confidence, difficulties in establishing interpersonal
communication, and dependency (which is concealed beneath
a facade of self-confidence and strong masculinity).

The growth of drinking during the Soviet period is also
connected with the economic deprivation of the majority of
the Soviet population, the suppression of the personality,
private initiative, and spiritual freedom. These produce
a growth of alienation, dissatisfaction, feelings of
insecurity, anger, and increasing escapist tendencies.
Finally, drinking--especially among young people--reflects
the need to create new tensions to substitute for the
loss of meaning in life and to avoid boredom.

The concept of alcoholism as a disease resembling drug
addiction is now shared more or less by Soviet and American
medical circles. However, the moralistic approach is still
very widespread among the authorities and public opinion,
which often demand censure and punishment for the alcoholic.

Although both countries are making definite efforts in the area of alcoholism prevention, these measures are inadequate. In the Soviet Union in particular, governmental measures attempting to curtail the production of "hard" beverages, increase the cost of alcohol, limit the places and times of sale, punish those who produce home-distilled "samogon," and institute compulsory treatment of alcoholics manifesting antisocial behavior have proved ineffective. The Soviet Union is making a greater attempt than the United States to utilize the mass media and social pressure against alcoholics with antisocial behavior. However, in the Soviet Union there is no national temperance movement, and the official "antialcohol propaganda" is received skeptically and is unable to alter positive attitudes toward drinking. On the other hand, the Soviet government has an interest in selling alcoholic beverages, and therefore the preventive measures that are undertaken are inconsistent. In both countries appropriate educational work with youth is insufficiently carried out.

Among the achievements of the American system of controlling alcoholism, the activity of the AA and the clergy and the existence of social workers and counselling programs must be included.

The organization of the Soviet medical system for the treatment of alcoholics has a number of advantages over the American system. However, in both countries the quality of medical care is not equal for various social groups in urban and rural areas.

The majority of Soviet and American psychiatrists and physicians consider no single form of treatment suitable in every case and support a multidisciplinary approach to therapy. In practice, however, frequently and unfortunately the same stereotyped methods are applied, and individualized and multidisciplinary approaches are ignored.

In the United States, group psychotherapy is used more extensively, while in the Soviet Union treatment by aversive therapy, hypnosis, so-called "rational" psychotherapy, and autogenic training (relaxation) are widespread. Despite the didactic and paternalistic tendencies in Soviet psychotherapy, it has recently moved closer to its American counterpart.

Medical methods of treatment in both countries are even more similar. In the area of medical care, the insufficient number of qualified medical personnel devoted entirely to treatment and after-care, the insufficient intercommunication between medical, government, social, and educational institutions, and also the limited funds devoted to research and the search for new, effective methods of treatment remain the main problems.

BIBLIOGRAPHY

1. Pryzhov, Ivan, Istoriya kabakov v Rossii (The History of Taverns in Russia), St. Petersburg - Moscow: M. O. Vol'f, 1868.

2. Bol'shaya meditsinskaya entsiklopediya (The Great Medical Encyclopedia), Vol. 1 (1956), col. 727, fig. 1.

3. Narodnoe Khozyaistvo SSSR v 1962 godu (The National Economy of the USSR in 1963). Moscow: "Statistika," 1963.

4. Narodnoe Khozyaistvo SSSR v 1973 godu (The National Economy of the USSR in 1973). Moscow: "Statistika," 1974.

5. Treml, Vladimir G. "Production and Consumption of Alcoholic Beverages in the USSR: A Statistical Study," Quart. Journ. Stud. Alc., Vol. 36, No. 3, March 1975, 285-320.

6. Sovetskaya Torgovlya v 1972 godu: Statisticheskii Sbornik (Soviet Trade in 1972: Collection of Statistics), Moscow, 1973.

7. Narodnoe Khozyaistvo Latviiskoi SSR v 1972 godu (The National Economy of the Latvian SSR in 1972). Riga, 1973.

8. As quoted in V. Bykov, Ekonomika i organizatsiya promyshlennogo proizvodstva (The Economics and Organization of Industrial Manufacture), 1974, No. 4, 49-50.

9. Strel'chuk, I. V., Klinika i lechenie narkomanii (Clinical Traits and Treatment of Addictions), Moscow: Medgiz, 1956.

10. Balyakin, V. A., Toksikologiya i ekspertiza alkogol'nogo op'yaneniya (Toxicology and Expertise of Alcoholic Intoxication), Moscow: Meditsina, 1962.

11. Tkachevskii, Yu. M., Prestupnost' i alkogolizm (Crime and Alcoholism), Moscow: Znanie, 1966.

12. Sakharov, A. V., O lichnosti prestupnika i prichinakh prestupnosti v SSSR (The Personality of the Criminal and the Causes of Crime in the USSR), Moscow: Yuridicheskaya Literatura, 1961.

13. Alkogolizm - put' k prestupleniyu (Alcoholism - The Road to Crime), Moscow: Yuridicheskaya Literatura, 1965.

14. Segal, B. M., Alkogolizm: klinicheskie, sotsial'no-psikhologicheskie i biologicheskie problemy (Alcoholism: Clinical, Socio-Psychological, and Biological Problems), Moscow: Meditsina, 1961.

15. Problemy sudebnoi psikhiatrii (The Problems of Forensic Psychiatry), Vol. IX, 372, Moscow: Yuridicheskaya Literatura, 1961.

16. Rozhnov, V. E., Po sledam zelenogo zmeya (Tracking the Green Serpent), Moscow: Voennoe Izdatel'stvo, 1969.

17. Banshchikov, V. M., Alkogolizm i ego vred dlya zdorov'ya cheloveka (Alcoholism and Its Dangers to Human Health), Moscow, 1958.

18. Zaigraev, G. G., "O nekotorykh problemakh bor'by s p'yanstvom " ("Some Problems of the Fight against Drunkenness"), Voprosy preduprezhdeniya prestupnosti, Moscow: Yuridicheskaya Literatura, 1966.

19. Tkachevskii, Yu. M., Pravda, March 29, 1969.

20. Kachaev, A. K., "O nekotorykh somaticheskikh i
     psikhicheskikh korrelyatsiyakh v patogeneze
     alkogol'nykh rasstroistv " ("Some Somatic and Mental
     Correlations and the Pathogenesis of Alcoholic
     Disorders"), Materialy V vsesoyuznogo s"ezda nevro-
     patologov i psikhiatrov (Proceedings of the Fifth
     All-Union Congress of Neurologists and Psychiatrists),
     Vol. 3, 411-414, Moscow, 1969.

21. Goldovskaya, T. I., Puti i metody izucheniya nervno-
     psikhicheskoi zabolevaemosti (Methods of Examination
     of Mental Morbidity), Moscow: Gos. Institut
     Psikhiatrii, 1964.

22. Zabolevaemost' gorodskogo naseleniya i normativy
     lechebno-profilakticheskoi pomoshchi (Morbidity of
     the Urban Population and Norms of Preventive and
     Medical Care), I. D. Bogatyrev, ed., Moscow:
     Meditsina, 1967.

23. Simonov, P. K., Printsipy organizatsii protivoakogol'noi
     raboty v somaticheskoi i psikhonevrologicheskoi seti
     (The Principles of Organization of Treatment of
     Alcoholics in the General and Mental Health Services),
     I. Lukomskii, ed., Moscow: Gos. Institut Psikhiatrii,
     1963, 377-383.

24. Dorsht, A. Ya., "K voprosu o strukture nervno-
     psikhicheskoi zabolevaemosti gorodskogo i sel'skogo
     naseleniya " ("The Structure of the Neuro-Psychiatric
     Morbidity of the Urban and Rural Population"),
     Voprosy organizatsii psikhonevrologicheskoi pomoshchi
     i psikhoprofilaktiki (Organization of Psychiatric
     Service and Prevention), Stavropol: Meditsinskii
     Institut, 1962.

25. Strel'chuk, I. V., Ostraya i khronicheskaya
     intoksikatsiya alkogolem (Acute and Chronic Alcohol
     Intoxication), Moscow: Meditsina, 1973.

26. Segal, B. M., "Rol' nevrozov v geneze alkogolizma,"
     ("The Role of Neuroses in the Origin of Alcoholism")
     Zhurnal nevropatologii i psikhiatrii imeni S. S.
     Korsakova, 2, 1967, 246-253.

27. Segal, B. M., L. N. Nerobkova, and S. V. Rybalkina,
     "Vlechenie" k alkogolyu pri stimulyatsii yader
     gipotalamusa u krys ("Craving" for Alcohol in Rats
     after Stimulation of the Hypothalamic Nuclei),
     Zhurnal vysshei nervnoi deyatel'nosti imeni I. P.
     Pavlova, XIX, No. 4, 1969, 688-691.

28. Segal, B. M., M. V. Kushnarev, et al. "Alcoholism and
     the Disruption of the Activity of Deep Cerebral
     Structures," Quart. J. Stud. Alc., Vol. 31, No. 3,
     1970, 587-601.

29. Gurevich, M. L. Uchebnik psikhiatrii (Psychiatric
     Textbook), Moscow: Medgiz, 1949.

30. Gilyarovskii, V. A., Psikhiatriya (Psychiatry),
     Moscow: Medgiz, 1954.

31. Popov, E. A., Intoksikatsionnye psikhozy: Uchebnik
     psikhiatrii (Intoxicational Psychoses: Psychiatric
     Textbook), Kerbikov, O. V. et al., eds., Moscow:
     Medgiz, 1958.

32. Zhislin, S. G., Ob alkogol'nykh rasstroistvakh
     (Alcoholic Disorders), Voronezh, 1935.

33. Vedomosti verkhovnogo soveta RSFSR, No. 10 (804),
     March 7, 1974, 285-288.

34. Entin, G. M., Prakticheskoe rukovodstvo po lecheniyu
     alkogolizma (Manual on the Treatment of Alcoholism),
     Moscow: Meditsina, 1972.

35. Entin, G. M., Lechenie alkogolizma v usloviyakh
     uchrezhdenii obshchemeditsinskoi seti (Treatment of
     Alcoholism in the Network of General Medicine),
     Moscow: Meditsina, 1967.

36. Alkogolizm i toksikomanii (Alcoholism and Addictions),
     D. Fedotov, Ed., Moscow: Moskovskii Institut
     Psikhiatrii, 1968.

37. Zenevitch, G. V., S. S. Libikh, Psikhoterapiya
     Alkogolizma (The Psychotherapy of Alcoholism),
     Moscow: Meditsina, 1965.

38. Rozhnov, V. E., Lektsii po psikhoterapii (Lectures on Psychotherapy), Moscow: Ministerstvo Zdravookhraneniya SSSR, 1971.

39. Segal, B. M., "Metod autogennoi trenirovki v sisteme psikhoterapii pri alkogolizme " ("Autogenic Training and Psychotherapy of Alcoholism") Voprosy psikhoterapii, V. Banshchikov and M. Lebedinskii, eds., Moscow: Vsesoyuznoe obshchestvo nevropatologov i psikhiatrov, 1966, 201-202.

40. "Alkogolizm i alkogol'nye psikhozy " ("Alcoholism and Alcoholic Psychoses"), Sbornik rabot, I. Lukomskii, ed., Moscow: Gos. Institut Psikhiatrii, 1963.

41 Patogenez i klinika alkogol'nykh zabolevanii (The Pathogenesis and Clinical Features of Alcohol Disorders), I. Lukomskii, ed., Moscow: Vsesoyuznoe soveshchanie, 1970.

42. Alkogolizm i alkogol'nye psikhozy (Alcoholism and Alcohol Psychoses), Vol. 2, Omsk: Meditsinskii Institut, 1970.

43. Klinicheskie problemy alkogolizma (Clinical Problems of Alcoholism), G. Zenevich, ed., Moscow: Meditsina, 1974.

44. Problemy alkogolizma (Problems of Alcoholism), Vol. 3 and 4, G. Morozov, ed., Moscow: Ministerstvo Zdravookhraneniya, 1973-1974.

45. Lukomskii, I. I., G. M. Entin, Voprosy organizatsii bor'by s alkogolizmom (Organization of Care for Alcoholism), Moscow, Meditsina.

46. Portnov, A. A., I. N. Pyatnitskaya, Klinika alkogolizma (Clinical Traits of Alcoholism), Moscow: Meditsina, 1973.

47. New York Times, September 30, 1975.

48. Efron, V., M. Keller, and C. Gurioli, Statistics on Consumption of Alcohol and on Alcoholism, New Brunswick: Rutgers Center of Alcohol Studies, 1974.

49. Cahalan, D., I. H. Cisin, and H. M. Crossley,
     "American Drinking Practices: A National Survey of
     Behavior and Attitudes," Rutgers Center Alc. Stud.
     No. 6 (1969), New Brunswick.

50. Cahalan, D., and I. H. Cisin, "American Drinking
     Practices: Summary of Findings from a National
     Probability Sample. Measurement of Massed vs.
     Spaced Drinking," Quart. J. Stud. Alc. 29, (1968),
     642-656.

51. Cahalan, D., Problem Drinkers, San Francisco:
     Josey-Boss, 1970.

52. Kimes, W. T., S. C. Smith and R. E. Maher, Alcohol and
     Drug Abuse in South Carolina High Schools, Columbia,
     S. C.: South Carolina Dept. of Education, 1969.

53. Hodges, E. H., High School Drinking in Georgia: Report,
     Atlanta: Georgia Dept. of Public Health, 1971.

54. New York Times, August 3, 1975.

55. Sakharov, A. D., My Country and the World, Alfred A.
     Knopf, 1975.

56. California's Alcoholism: Problems and Resources.,
     Division of Alcoholic Rehabilitation, State Dept. of
     Public Health, 1964.

57. Wolfgang, M. and R. B. Strohm, "The Relationship
     between Alcohol and Criminal Homicide," Quart. J.
     Stud. Alcohol., 17: 1956: 411-425.

58. Mac Cormick, A. H., "Correctional Views on Alcohol,
     Alcoholism, and Crime," Crime and Delinquency,
     9:1963: 15-28.

59. Tinklenberg, J. R., "Alcohol and Violence,"
     Alcoholism: Progress in Research and Treatment,
     P. G. Bourne, R. Fox, eds., Academic Press, 1973,
     195-210.

60. Fox, R. "The Effects of Alcoholism on Children,"
     Proceedings of the Fifth International Congress on
     Psychotherapy, 1963.

61. Jackson, J. K., "Alcoholism and the Family," Society, Culture, and Drinking Patterns, D. J. Pittman and Ch. R. Snyder, eds., Carbondale, Ill.: S. Illinois Univ. Press, 1973, 422-492.

62. Fine, E. W., "Alcoholic Family: Dynamics and their Effect on Children," Alcoholism Digest, Vol. IV, No. 7, July, 1975, vi-ix.

63. Bailey, M. B. and B. Leach, Alcoholics Anonymous: Pathways to Recovery. A Study of 1058 Members of the A. A. Membership in New York City, New York: NCA, 1965.

64. Pell, S. and C. A. D'Alonzo, "The Prevalence of Chronic Disease Among Problem Drinkers," Archives of Environmental Health, May 1968, Vol. 16, 679-684.

65. New York Times, May 3, 1975.

66. Mulford, H. A., and D. Miller, "Drinking in Iowa, II: The Extent of Drinking and Selected Socio-cultural Categories," Quart. J. Stud. Alcohol, 21: 1960: 260-391.

67. Knupfer, G., "Characteristics of Abstainers: A Comparison of Drinkers and Non-Drinkers in a Large California City," Report No. 3: California Drinking Practice Study., Berkeley, Cal.: Division of Alcoholic Rehabilitation, Dept. of Public Health, Nov. 1961.

68. Bales, R. F., "The Fixation Factor," Alcoholic-Addiction: An Hypothesis Derived from a Comparative Study of Irish and Jewish Social Norms., Doctoral Dissertation, Harvard University, 1944.

69. Thorner, I., "Ascetic Protestantism and Alcoholism," Psychiatry, 16: 1953, 167-176.

70. Scolnick, J. H., "Religious Affiliation and Drinking Behavior," Quart. J. Stud. Alc., 19: 1958: 452-470.

71. Lolli, G., E. Serianni, G. M. Golder, and P. Luzzatto-Fegiz, Alcohol in Italian Culture, New Haven: Publications Division, Yale Center of Alcohol Studies, and Glencoe, Ill.: Free Press, 1958.

72. Chafetz, M. E., and H. W. Demone, Alcoholism and
     Society, New York: Oxford Univ. Press, 1962.

73. Bales, R. F., "Attitudes Toward Drinking in the Irish
     Culture," Society, Culture, and Drinking Patterns,
     D. J. Pittman and Ch. R. Snyder, Eds., Carbondale,
     Ill.: Southern Illinois Univ. Press, 1973, 157-187.

74. Snyder, Ch. R., "Culture and Jewish Sobriety: The
     Ingroup-Outgroup Factor," Society, Culture, and
     Drinking Patterns, D. J. Pittman and Ch. R. Snyder,
     Eds., Carbondale, Ill.: Southern Illinois Univ.
     Press, 1973, 188-225.

75. Straus, R. and S. D. Bacon, Drinking in College, New
     Haven: Yale Univ. Press, 1953.

76. Hooton, C. What Shall We Say about Alcohol?,New York:
     Abingdon Press, 1960.

77. Albrecht, G. L., "The Alcoholism Process: A Social
     Learning Viewpoint," Alcoholism: Progress in Research
     and Treatment, P. G. Bourne and R. Fox, eds., New
     York: Academic Press, 1973, 11-42.

78. Hyman, M. M., "Accident Vulnerability and Blood Alcohol
     Concentrations in Drivers by Demographic Characteristics,
     Quart. J. Stud. Alc. Suppl. No. 4, 1968, 34-57.

79. Barchha, R., M. A. Stewart, and S. B. Cuze, "Prevalence
     of Alcoholism among General Hospital Ward Patients,"
     Amer. J. Psychiatry, 125, 1968, 681-684.

80. Bourne, P. G., "Alcoholism in the Urban Negro Population
     Alcoholism: Progress in Research and Treatment, P. G.
     Bourne and R. Fox, eds., New York: Academic Press,
     1973, 211-226.

81   Pittman, D. J., "Drinking and Alcoholism in American
     Society," Alcoholism: The Total Treatment Approach,
     R. J. Catanzaro, ed., Springfield, Ill.: Ch. C. Thomas,
     1974, 70-79.

82. Myerson, A., "Alcohol: A Study of Social Ambivalency,"
     Quart. J. Stud. Alcohol, 1: 13-20.

83. Dollard, J., "Drinking Mores of the Social Classes,"
    Alcohol: Science and Society, New Haven: Journal of
    Studies on Alcohol, 1945.

84. Lawrence, J. J., M. A. Maxwell, "Drinking and Socio-
    Economic Status," Society, Culture, and Drinking
    Patterns, D. J. Pittman and Ch. R. Snyder, eds.,
    Carbondale, Ill.: Southern Illinois University
    Press, 1973, 141-145.

85. Stone, G. P., "Drinking Styles and Status
    Arrangements," Society, Culture, and Drinking Patterns,
    D. J. Pittman and Ch. R. Snyder, eds., Carbondale,
    Ill.: Southern Illinois University Press, 1973,
    121-140.

86. Bales, R. F., "Cultural Differences in Rates of
    Alcoholism," Quart. J. Stud. Alcohol, 6 (March, 1946),
    400-499.

87. Roebuck, J. B., R. G. Kessler, The Etiology of
    Alcoholism, Springfield, Ill.: Ch. C. Thomas, 1972.

88. Straus, R., "Alcohol and Society," Psychiatric Annals,
    3:10, Oct., 1973.

89. "Posle bala "("After the Ball"), Sovetskaya Molodezh
    (Soviet Youth), No. 216, 1975.

90. Maddox, G. L., "Drinking Prior to College," The
    Domesticated Drug: Drinking Among Collegians, G. L.
    Maddox, ed., New Haven: College and Univ. Press, 1971.

91. Maddox, G. L., "Teenage Drinking in the United States,"
    Society, Culture, and Drinking Patterns, D. J. Pittman
    and Ch. R. Snyder, eds., Carbondale, Ill.: Southern
    Illinois University Press, 1973, 230-245.

92. Eisenstadt, S. N., From Generation to Generation: Age
    Groups and Social Structure, Glencoe, Ill.: Free Press,
    1956.

93. Erikson, E. H., Identity, Youth, and Crisis, New York:
    W. W. Norton and Co., 1968.

94. Komsomol'skaya pravda (Komsomol Truth), No. 48, 1975.

95. Segal, B. M., "Drinking and Alcoholism in Russia," Psychiatric Opinion, Vol. 12, No. 9, 1975, 21-29.

96. Kopyt, N. Ya., V. G. Zaposhchenko, O. Chekaida. Metodicheskie podkhody k izucheniyu rasprostranennosti alkogolizma na promyshlennom predpriyatii ("Methodological Approach to the Analysis of the Prevalence of Alcoholism in a Factory"), Zdravookhranenie Rossiiskoi Federatsii, No. 8, 1972, 13-16.

97. Alcoholism: The Total Treatment Approach, R. J. Catanzaro, ed., Springfield, Ill.: Ch. C. Thomas, 1974, 5-25.

98. Losskii, N. O., Kharakter russkogo naroda (The Character of the Russian People), Frankfurt-Main: Possev-Verlag, 1957.

99. Berdyaev, N., Russkaya ideya (The Russian Idea), Paris: YMCA-Press, 1971.

100. Klyuchevskii, V., Kurs russkoi istorii, Vol. 1, Lecture XVII (Course of Russian History), Sotsekhiz, 1937.

101. Chekhov, A. P., Izbrannye proizvedeniya (Selected Works), Vol. III., Moscow: Khudozhestvennaya literatura, 1964, p. 144.

102. Ibid., p. 7.

103. Bunin, I. A., Sobranie sochinenii (Collection of Works), Vol. II, Moscow: Pravda, 1956, p. 9.

104. Veresaev, V. V., Povesti i rasskazy (Tales and Stories), Kishinev: Gosizdat, 1958, p. 3.

105. Bunin, I. A., Sobranie sochinenii (Collection of Works), Vol. III, Moscow: Pravda, 1956, p. 147.

106. Menninger, K. A., Man Against Himself, New York: Harcourt, Brace, 1938.

107. Freud, S., Three Contributions to the Theory of Sex, Standard Ed., London: Hogarth, 1953, Vol. 7.

108. Abraham, K. L., Psychological Relations Between Sexuality and Alcoholism, Selected Papers, London: Hogarth, 1927.

109. Adler, A., "The Individual Psychology of the Alcoholic Patient," J. Crim. Psychopath., 3:74-77, 1941.

110. McCord, W., and J. McCord, "A Longitudinal Study of the Personality of Alcoholics," Society, Culture and Drinking Patterns, D. J. Pittman and Ch. R. Snyder, eds., Carbondale, Ill.: Southern Illinois University Press, 1973, 413-430.

111. Lolli, G., "Alcoholism as a Disorder of the Love Disposition," Quart. J. Stud. Alcohol, 17, 1950, 96-107.

112. Lissasky, E., The Etiology of Alcoholism: The Role of Psychological Predisposition, Quart. J. Stud. Alcohol, 21, 314-343, 1960.

113. The Person with Alcoholism, F. A. Seixas, et al., eds., Vol. 233, New York Academy of Sciences, 1974.

114. Blane, H. T., The Personality of the Alcoholic: Guises of Dependency, New York: Harper and Row, 1968.

115. Hayman, M., Alcoholism. Mechanism and Management, Springfield, Ill.: Ch. C. Thomas, 1966.

116. Smith, H., The Russians, Quadrangle/The New York Times Book Co., 1976.

117. Bulgakov, M., Sobach'e serdtse (Heart of the Dog), Harcourt Brace Jovanovich, New York, 1968.

118. Zoshchenko, M., Rasskazy (Stories), Frankfurt/Main: Possev-Verlag, 1971.

119. Pomerants, G., Neopublikovannoe (Unpublished Material), Frankfurt/Main: Possev-Verlag, 1972.

120. Maksimov, V., Sem' dnei tvoreniya (Seven Days of Creation), Paris: YMCA-Press, 1971.

121. Shukshin, V., Kharaktery (Characters), Moscow: Sovremennik, 1973.

122. Lipatov, V., Dve Povesti (Two Stories), Molodaya gvardiya, 1972.

123. Horton, D., "The Functions of Alcohol in Primitive Societies: A Cross-Cultural Study," Quart. J. Stud. Alcohol , 4, 1943, 199-320.

124. Field, P. B., "A New Cross-Cultural Study of Drunkenness," Society, Culture, and Drinking Patterns, D. J. Pittman and Ch. R. Snyder, eds., Carbondale, Ill.: Southern Illinois University Press, 1973, 48-74.

125. Allport, G. W., Pattern and Growth in Personality, New York: Holt, 1961.

126. Kalant, H., "Some Recent Physiological and Biochemical Investigations on Alcohol and Alcoholism," Quart. J. Stud. Alcohol , 23 (March, 1962), 52-93.

127. Alcoholism: Progress in Research and Treatment, P. G. Bourne and R. Fox, eds., New York: Academic Press, 1973, 227-243.

128. Medical Consequences of Alcoholism, F. A. Seixas, K. Williams, and S. Eggleston, eds., New York: New York Academy of Sciences, 1975.

129. The Biology of Alcoholism. Volumes I-III. Kissin, B., ed., N.Y.-London: Plenum Press.

130. Ullman, A. D., "First Drinking Experience as Related to Age and Sex," Society, Culture, and Drinking Patterns, D. J. Pittman and Ch. R. Snyder, eds., Carbondale, Ill.: Southern Illinois University Press, 1973, 259-266.

131. Fox, R., "A Multidisciplinary Approach to the Treatment of Alcoholism," Amer. J. Psychiat., 123:7, Jan. 1967: 769-778.

132. Jellinek, E. M., "Phases in the Drinking Motives of Alcoholics," Quart. J. Stud. Alc., 7: 1946: 1-88.

133. Isbell, H., H. F. Fraser, A. Wikler, R. E. Belleville, and A. J. Eisenman, "An Experimental Study of the Etiology of 'Rum Fits' and Delirium Tremens," Quart. J. Stud. Alcohol, 16: 1: 1955: 1-33.

134. Victor, M., and R. D. Adams, "The Effect of Alcohol on the Nervous System," Res. Publ. Association of Nervous and Mental Diseases, 32: 1956: 526-573.

135. Forum: The Prevention of Alcoholism, F. A. Seixas, ed., New York: National Council on Alcoholism, 1971.

136. Manual on Alcoholism, Chicago: Amer. Med. Assoc., 1973.

137. Wallerstein, R. S., Hospital Treatment of Alcoholism, Menninger Clinic Monograph Series No. 11, New York: Basic Books, 1957.

138. Glasscote, R. M., et al., The Treatment of Alcoholism: A Study of Programs and Problems, Washington, D. C.: American Psychiatric Association, 1967.

139. Connor, W. D., Deviance in Soviet Society: Crime, Delinquency, and Alcoholism, New York and London: Columbia University Press, 1972.

140. American Sociology, T. Parsons, ed., New York and London: Basic Books, Inc., 1968.

141. Lebedinskii, M. S., Ocherki psikhoterapii (Essays on Psychotherapy), Moscow: Meditsina, 1971.

142. Voprosy kliniki i psikhoterapii alkogolizma i nevrozov (Clinical Picture and Psychotherapy of Alcoholism and Neuroses), V. Rozhnov, ed., Moscow: Ministerstvo Zdravookhraneniya, 1974.

143. Libikh, S. S., Kollektivnaya psikhoterapiya nevrozov (Collective Psychotherapy of Neuroses), Leningrad: Meditsina, 1973.

144. Curley, J., "How a Therapist Can Use A.A.," The Person with Alcoholism, F. A. Seixas, R. Cadoret, S. Eggleston, eds., N. Y. Academy of Sciences, 1974: 137.

ADDENDUM

A Multidisciplinary Study of Alcoholism

in the Soviet Union

Various concepts of the etiology of alcoholism were analyzed by the author and his coworkers between 1954-1967 (1). A total of 1703 alcoholics were investigated in Moscow hospitals and outpatient clinics.

The analysis showed, first of all, that no significant difference existed between alcoholics and nonalcoholics in their social, economic and educational background (1). The influence of sociopsychological factors (drinking patterns, attitudes of family) was very significant. In 70% of the cases the parents tolerated "moderate" drunkenness and in 10% hard drinking was accepted. Still more striking data were acquired in a study of "friends," where heavy drinking was the norm in 53% of the cases and "moderate" drinking in 43% (1, 2). The influence of social group was most evident in teen-aged drinkers.

The tranquillizing effect of alcohol was sought by 33%, stimulating and euphoric effects by 20% of all cases (1).

An epidemiological study has shown that a prealcoholic state, accompanied by expressed neurotic and psychopathic symptoms, varied from 19.8 to 26.1% (in different groups). But most of the other patients were so-called "persons of external norms" (Luxenburger). For them there exists only "the danger of disintegration" under stress. In other words, "real" neurotics become alcoholics relatively rarely (3). At the same time in more than half of the cases (52.5%) there were signs of an "unhappy childhood" (lack of a parent, etc.). Homosexual tendencies were found in 4% of male and in 2% of female cases. Such factors as a domineering mother and oral habits did not correlate with the rapid start of alcoholism. Nevertheless, early weaning of those in the group, along with rapid development of a physical dependency, was statistically significant (1, 3). The important role of suppressed aggressive and destructive impulses, hostility and anger, and such traits as dependency, introvertiveness, a sense of guilt, anxiety and depression, especially during the acute withdrawal period, as well as maladjustment and sexual problems, was determined by psychological tests (TAT, MMPI). All patients refused to face the fact of their alcoholism for many years, using the defensive mechanisms of denial, rationalization and projection of the blame onto their spouses or circumstances.

A premorbid failure of the autonomic and endocrine systems was observed in 13.5% of the cases. But these insufficiencies in patients with an early history of alcoholism were twice those of patients with late development of alcoholism. Moreover, the possibility of the existence of subtle and latent deviations must be kept in mind (1). A craving for alcohol was magnified by injuries to the brain (p < 0.01). Clinical study showed that alcoholism is a special progredient disease, whose main clinical traits are various forms of a pathological craving for alcohol (1). The first stage occurs after 5 to 6 years of alcohol abuse and lasts for 2 to 3 years. It is characterized by excessive drinking with loss of control over the use of alcohol.

A clear withdrawal syndrome with expressed physical and psychological dependency (addiction) and considerable disruption of social and family relations, as well as somatic disorders, are seen in the second stage (chronic alcoholism). In this stage all other symptoms of a changed reaction toward alcohol are clearly manifested: changes of tolerance, type and system of drinking, etc. This phase develops 6 to 9 years after the beginning of the systematic consumption of alcohol and lasts for a period of from 3 to 5 years.

The third stage is distinguished by severe periodic (dipsomanic-like) bouts consequent upon the grave physical dependency, as well as deterioration and psychoses. It sets in from approximately 7 to 12 years after the beginning of systematic drinking. Of course, this is merely a general outline of this process, which can be stopped at every stage (4, 5).

Like other authors, we determined that alcoholism leads to functional and then organic disturbances: encephalopathies, liver cirrhosis, pancreatitis,

myocardiodystrophia (6). Local cerebral hypertension,
asymmetry and paradoxic responses of autonomic and vascular
systems were seen (7, 8). Biochemical and endocrinologic
data indicated inhibition of radioiodine absorption by the
thyroid gland, depletion of the activity of the hypophysial-
adrenal system, dysfunction of insular and sexual glands,
and disruption of water, mineral and carbohydrate metabolism
during the acute withdrawal period (1, 8, 9). A significant
decrease in the serotonin and catecholamine levels in the
blood was reported (1, 8, 10, 11). This testifies to the
dysfunction of both the ergotropic and the trophotropic
systems, especially in conjunction with the abstinence
syndrome.

A high percentage of desynchronized curves with slow
flat oscillations has been seen in electroencephalograms
(EEG) during the severe withdrawal period. Polyrhythmic
alpha activity and paroxysmal discharges of theta and of
spiked waves prevalent in parieto-central and frontal regions
were seen often. Patients in the intial stage of alcoholism
were characterized by a tendency toward normalization of
reactivity during afferent stimulation and epinephrine
loading. In severe cases (the third stage) afferent stimulation and epinephrine effected a decrease in EEG reactivity. Spontaneous oscillations of skin potential and gal-
vanic skin response amplitude were increased (1, 8, 12).
The polymorphous character of the above disorders indicates
violations of the homeostatic and adaptive functions controlled by the deep structures of the brain. This hypothesis
is confirmed by the fact that alcoholic disorders, especially the abstinence syndrome, are very close to those observed
in patients with organic damage of the reticulo-hypothalamic
limbic structures (1, 8, 12). Experiments with rats have
revealed the close relations between "craving" for alcohol
and the functional state of the hypothalamic system. After
the stimulation of the "punishment system," a craving for
alcohol was initiated. When the "reinforcement system" was
stimulated and self-stimulated and reactions of food consuming and sexual nature were observed, alcoholic consumption
either decreased or ceased entirely (1, 13).

Thus, our epidemiological, clinical, laboratory and
experimental data confirmed on the one hand that there are
several social and psychological factors predisposing a
person to heavy drinking. But the development of alcohol

addiction requires that these factors be accompanied by
particular autonomic and biochemical changes, both
hereditary and acquired. On the other hand, these data
permitted us to offer a concept of alcohol disorders as
a result of dysfunction of limbic and reticulo-hypothalamic
structures.

ADDENDUM

BIBLIOGRAPHY

1. Segal, B. M., Alkogolizm: Klinicheskie, sotsial'no-
    psikhologicheskie i biologicheskie problemy
    (Alcoholism: Clinical, Socio-Psychological, and
    Biological Problems). Moscow: Meditsina, 1967.

2. Segal, B. M., Drozdov, E. S., "Mikrosotsial'naya
    sreda i sotsial'naya readaptatsiya pri alkogolizme "
    ("Microsocial Environment and Social Readaptation in
    Alcoholism"), In: Vosstanovitel'naya terapiya i
    sotsial'no-trudovaya readaptatsiya (Rehabilitation
    Therapy and Social-Occupational Readaptation), E. S.
    Averbukh, Ed., Leningrad: Institut imeni Bekhtereva,
    1965, pp. 293-296.

3. Segal, B. M., "Nevrozy i alkogolizm " ("Neuroses and
    Alcoholism"), In: Pogranichnye sostoyaniya
    (Borderline Conditions), O. V. Kerbikov, ed., Moscow:
    Ministerstvo Zdravookhraneniya, 1965, 325-329.

4. Segal, B. M., "O nekotorykh psikhopatologicheskikh
    osobennostyakh alkogol'nogo abstinentnogo sindroma "
    ("Some Psychopathological Features of the Alcohol
    Withdrawal Syndrome"), In: Problemy sotsial'noy
    i klinicheskoy psikhonevrologii (Problems of Social
    and Clinical Psychoneurology), L. L. Rokhlin, ed.,
    Moscow: Moskovskii Institut Psikhiatrii, 1961,
    245-251.

5. Segal, B. M., Urakov, I. G., "Seksual'nye rasstroistva
    pri alkogolizme " ("Sexual Disorders in Alcoholism"),
    In: Aktual'nye Problemy Seksopatologii (Relevant
    Problems of Sexual Pathology), D. D. Fedotov, ed.,
    Moscow: Moskovskii Institut Psikhiatrii, 1967,
    322-340.

6. Segal, B. M., Urakov, I. G., "Nevrozy, nevrozopodobnye
    sostoyaniya i funktsional'nye somaticheskie
    narusheniya pri alkogolizme " (Neuroses, Neurosis-like
    Conditions, and Functional Somatic Disorders in
    Alcoholism), In: Nevrozy i somaticheskie rasstroistva
    (Neuroses and Somatic Disorders), M. M. Kabanov, ed.,
    Leningrad: Ministerstvo Zdravookhraneniya, 1965, 76-78.

7. Segal, B. M., Urakov, I. G., "Rol' vegetativnykh i
    somaticheskikh narushenii v klinike i patogeneze
    alkogolizma " ("The Role of Vegetative and Somatic
    Disorders in the Clinical Picture and Pathogenesis of
    Alcoholism"), In: D. D. Fedotov (ed.), Alkogolizm i
    toksikomanii (Alcoholism and Addictions). Moscow:
    Moskovskii Institut Psikhiatrii, 1968. Pp. 79-84.

8. Segal, B. M., Kushnarev, V. M., et al., "Rol'
    dientsefal'noi patologii v strukture alkogol'nykh
    rasstroistv " ("The Role of Diencephalic Pathology in
    the Structure of Alcoholic Disorders"). In:
    Glubokie struktury golovnogo mozga i problemy psikhiatri
    (Deep Structures of the Brain and the Problems of
    Psychiatry), D. D. Fedotov, ed., Moscow: Moskovskii
    Institut Psikhiatrii, 1966, 216-223.

9. Segal, B. M., "O nekotorykh endokrinnykh narusheniyakh
    pri khronicheskom alkogolizme " ("Some Endocrine
    Disorders in Chronic Alcoholism"). In: Alkogolizm
    (Alcoholism), A. A. Portnov, ed., Moscow:
    Ministerstvo Zdravookhraneniya, 1959, 239-250.

10. Segal, B. M., Fedotov, D. D., Misionzhnik, E. Yu.
    "Affektivnye narusheniya pri alkogolizme i obmen
    katekholaminov " ("Affective Disorders in Alcoholism
    and Catecholamine Metabolism"). In: Trudy XXII
    nauchnoi sessii Ukrainskogo instituta nevropatologii i
    psikhiatrii (Proceedings of the 22nd Scientific
    Session of the Ukrainian Institute for Neuropathology
    and Psychiatry), Kharkov, 1965, 171-176.

11. Segal, B. M., Lando, L. I., "Alkogol'nyi abstinentnyi
    sindrom i obmen katekholaminov " ("Alcoholic Withdrawal
    Syndrome and Catecholamine Metabolism"). In: Klinika
    i lechenie alkogol'nykh zabolevanii (The Clinical
    Picture and Treatment of Alcoholic Illnesses), Moscow:
    Moskovskii Institut Psikhiatrii, 1966, 51-58.

12. Segal, B. M., Kushnarev, M. V., et al., "Alcoholism
     and the Disruption of the Activity of Deep Cerebral
     Structures," Quart. J. Stud. Alcohol , Vol. 31,
     No. 3, 1970, pp. 587-601.

13. Segal, B. M., Nerobkova, L. N., Rybalkina, S. V.,
     "Vlechenie k alkogolyu pri stimulyatsii yader
     gipotalamusa u krys " ("Craving for Alcohol in Rats
     When the Nuclei of the Hypothalamus are Stimulated").
     Zhurnal Vysshei Nervnoi Deyatel'nosti imeni I. P.
     Pavlova, (Pavlov Journal of Higher Nervous Activity),
     Vol. 19, No. 4, 1969, 688-691.

INVOLUNTARY HOSPITALIZATION IN THE USSR

Boris M. Segal

Russian Research Center

Harvard University, Cambridge, Massachusetts

Cases of the Soviet State's use of psychiatry in its struggle against political dissidents have received great publicity (1-16) and have provoked great indignation in the West (17-33). This indignation is largely incomprehensible to common Soviet people who know of more terrible instances of repression in the past (34).

If one views this problem in the broad sense, then one must recognize that the Soviet practice of the involuntary confinement of dissidents is in no way unprecedented or exceptional. In addition to its strictly medical function, psychiatry has a second, no less ancient function: the preservation of society. Viewed as a form of ideology, psychiatry should hinder the activity, actions, and even the thoughts that are abnormal and that threaten the stability and morals of the society. In an open society, controlled by laws and public opinion, this "spiritual-police" function of psychiatrists is kept to a minimum, although discussions about this role of psychiatry arise from time to time. But in a totalitarian state dominated by ideology, psychiatry is a completely legal means for controlling personality and for trying to prevent deviance from norms of behavior prescribed by the authorities.

Two equally mistaken ideas are common in evaluating the use of psychiatry in the Soviet Union for political and social aims. On the one hand, some skeptics deny the existence of repressive psychiatry (35). On the other hand, there is a tendency to overestimate the magnitude of such activity in the Soviet Union (36).

Thus, does the Soviet state really use this method of violence against its political opponents? And if so, then why do psychiatrists carry out directives of the authorities which are so incompatible with medical ethics? First of all let us adduce one example from Russian history. In 1836 Pyotr Chaadaev published "A philosophical letter," in which he sharply criticized Russia's historical role. This was a very explosive statement. It appeared during the reactionary reign of Nicholas I, when any original or liberal or "anti-patriotic" ideas were considered crimes. Official ideology at that time was "Orthodoxy, Autocracy, Nationalism." According to the chief of czarist secret police, Count Benkendorf, Russia had a splendid past; the present time was indeed admirable; and the future could not be predicted even in the most glowing terms. Therefore, the angered emperor pronounced Chaadaev insane.

Modern Soviet society is much more totalitarian than prerevolutionary Russian society and the Soviet authorities are much more intolerant to dissident points of view. Soviet psychiatry, like all other Soviet institutions, is completely subordinated to state (i.e., government) control. Chief doctors and other directors of psychiatric institutions are usually members of local soviets (organs of authority) along with other bureaucrats, among them officials of the KGB (Komitet Gosudarstvennoi Bezopasnosti [Committee on State Security], "the secret police"), the police, etc.

Mutual assistance among the entire leadership and the subordination of all to the "chief" (the first secretary of the district, city, or province Party committee) is the unwritten law of Soviet power. Therefore, when difficulties arise and the director of one agency turns to another for support, the latter generally is willing to help out a colleague. This support can mean placing an "active" dissident in a psychiatric hospital.

The following question arises. By what means can the forced hospitalization of a political dissident occur?

But before considering this question it is necessary to consider briefly the whole problem of involuntary hospitalization. The laws of involuntary hospitalization or institutionalization have been insufficiently studied and the larger public is unacquainted with them.

There are only vague references to involuntary hospitalization in the Criminal Codes of the Soviet republics. Instruction No. 04-14/32 promulgated by the Ministry of Public Health in 1962 states the following conditions for the institutionalization of a patient without his own consent or that of his relatives:

1. Psychomotor agitation with aggressive tendencies.

2. Anomalous behavior, brought about by mental disorders (hallucinations, delusions, etc.) if this behavior is connected with strong affective tension and a tendency to implementation.

3. Systematic paranoid syndrome with "progredient development" if it portends dangerous social behavior in the patient.

4. Hypochondriacal paranoiac states if they predispose to incorrect aggressive attitudes toward people or organizations.

A note to this instruction states that the patient may dissimulate pathological states and appear outwardly to have normal behavior. In addition the instruction emphasizes that not all, but only the most frequently encountered reasons for involuntary hospitalization are mentioned.

In 1969, this instruction was amplified by order No. 345-209 issued jointly by the Ministries of Public Health and Internal Affairs (the Soviet Police): "On the means of preventing socially dangerous acts by psychiatric patients." Both ministries said that the instruction of 1961 was not broad enough and ordered institutionalization not only for improper behavior, but also for potentially improper behavior and socially dangerous tendencies. The instruction does not define the psychiatric and legal grounds for hospitalization. These are cast in extremely vague terms, which gives the police and psychiatrists the opportunity to abuse psychiatric hospitals for political ends, since political speeches, demonstrations, passing manuscripts to the West and within Soviet literary circles can be considered socially dangerous.

Although the enforced institutionalization of healthy
people contravenes both the Soviet Criminal Code and international law, judges do not review complaints against such
actions.

The final decision on involuntary treatment is made by
a judge. It is based on a recommendation by a forensic
psychiatric commission named by the judge and prosecutor.
This commission can be composed of doctors from hospitals
or from outpatient clinics. The highest research and
training center for forensic psychiatry is the Serbskii
Institute which is under the jurisdiction of the Ministry
of Public Health, but is closely connected with the police
and the KGB. The accused does not know that he will be sent
before a commission and he is not informed of the results
of its deliberations "if his psychiatric condition makes
this impossible" (Article II, No. 84 of the Criminal Code
of the RSFSR). However, how and by whom this is ascertained
is not stated. The accused and his lawyer have no
possibility of influencing or disputing the commission's
findings. Often lawyers are not even provided, or
permitted to visit patients in mental hospitals. Each six
months, the commission is supposed to reconsider each case
of involuntary hospitalization, but this is rarely done.
And the commission can extend the period of hospitalization
beyond that decreed by the judge if the experts find that
the patient is not yet healthy. To avoid this, the patient
must confess that his thoughts and actions were incorrect.

Involuntary treatment takes place in special hospitals,
formerly called prison hospitals, and also in regular
psychiatric hospitals. The oldest and most terrible is the
Kazan Special Psychiatric Hospital. Later on, special
hospitals were established in Leningrad, Chernyakhovsk, and
Orel.

The regimen in these hospitals is more severe than in
regular psychiatric hospitals. The head doctor is a police
commandant. These hospitals are surrounded by barbed wire
and high fences, guarded by police. The doctors and
attendants are also police agents. Patients have even fewer
rights than typical mental patients. Meetings with close
relatives are permitted two or three times per month in the
presence of a guard; the patient's possessions and clothing
are searched; money and stationery are forbidden. Only

certain books are permitted; letters are censored and sent
only with the doctors' permission. The patient is allowed
to use the bathroom only a very limited number of times.

Patients are punished for refusing to see the doctor
or submit to treatment; such punishment may take the form of
a painful injection of sulfazine. Guards, many of whom are
criminals, frequently beat the patients. Patients are
required to work. Lights are kept on day and night, some
rooms are locked and patients are allowed out only to use
bathrooms and take walks. Before 1951, political prisoners
were separated from criminal prisoners, but now they are
kept together with murderers and run the risk of aggressive
attacks by psychotic patients. Involuntary treatment in
regular psychiatric hospitals, for example the Yakovenko
Hospital "Stolbovaya," is more lenient.

In my opinion, reports that dissidents are intention-
ally "driven to madness" through the use of some special
drugs lack foundation. The type of medication used is the
same as that used in all countries for the treatment of
paranoid states--chlorpromazine, stelazine, haloperidol,
and others. It is known that these drugs evoke unpleasant
sensations in the patient, disturbances of thinking, extra-
pyramidal symptoms, and other reactions. And it is true
that the attitude toward dissenters is in fact frequently
clear and coarse, but this corresponds to the general spirit
of Soviet closed psychiatric institutions (really prisons)
where measures of restraint have not yet been eliminated.

In the Soviet Union as in other countries, the
psychiatric system has been used to combat the antisocial
actions of people whose mental conditions are considered
pathological. Such persons can be tentatively divided into
three groups. The first consists of psychotic patients
who have committed violent criminal offenses (rape, murder,
etc.).

The second group consists for the most part of so-called
querulents. These are patients with so-called pathological
development of personality ("paranoiac developments"). The
activities of these persons are usually not directed against
the government but against individual people or institutions.
Their number is quite high. It is heterogeneous not only in
its nosological forms, but also in the character of the
querulents' antisocial actions.

Soviet psychiatrists often classify a wide range of
people as sick: those who want to reform political,
economic, or scientific institutions; fighters for justice;
"querulents" or "pathological slanderers" (who might defame
administrative officials). All these people write a great
number of complaints which besiege Party, state and
scientific institutions.* If their behavior becomes threatening or interferes with work, they are directed to
psychiatric examinations which frequently conclude with
institutionalization.

The psychic condition of these people goes beyond the
limits of normal, and their behavior is frequently absurd
indeed. However, this problem is more acute in the Soviet
Union than in the free world. Due to the high degree of
centralization, any active struggle with an administrative
person or organization is bound to expand into a struggle
with the system, which interrupts the bureaucratic order to
a greater degree than in an open society.

The last group is composed of persons with "anti-Soviet
delusions," those who act against the State. First of all,
this group includes patients whose paranoid ideas are anti-
Soviet. Due to the importance of the State in the life of
Soviet people, the frequency of such forms of expression
among psychotic patients is very high. Psychiatric
institutions have orders to hospitalize such patients as
soon as possible and not to release them without special
permission. It is curious that in the past, during Stalin's
terror, many psychotic patients were viewed as enemies of
the people and were imprisoned or shot.

But in recent times persons with rather doubtful cases
of mental illness have been included in this group of
patients. A tendency has arisen which is the opposite of
that which obtained under Stalin. The political basis for
this change can be found in the changes in Soviet society.
Under Stalin's heirs, mass terror and senseless repression
ceased. Party and state leaders are trying to avoid the

---

* Complaints literally flood all Soviet institutions. A
colossal staff of bureaucrats in a myriad of offices are
occupied with an endless review of and response to people's
grievances. They are obliged also to respond to
grievances from mental patients.

political measures which received widespread publicity and
which were condemned by Western public opinion. Therefore
the secret police (the KGB) has found itself in a difficult
position. On the one hand it is expected to be vigilant and
to conduct a struggle with anti-Soviet elements. On the
other hand in recent years the KGB has been subjected to
some measure of Party control and of legal restraint.
Therefore the secret police tries to use psychiatry for the
protection of the Soviet system.

Often when the KGB or other Party organs questioned
psychiatrists about the existence of mental disorders in a
particular dissenter, they frequently received positive
responses based on undefined criteria for mental illness.
In many cases one cannot clearly see a conscious evil design
of the KGB or psychiatrists. The former relies on the
conclusions of the latter. Meanwhile some psychiatrists
honestly believe that the dissidents are not mentally
healthy because their style of life and behavior do not
conform to "normal," well adapted behavior. Very few
psychiatrists "discover" mental illness only to serve the
authorities and to punish the liberals. But at the same
time one should not discount the desire of the authorities
to discredit their political opponents as "mad."

This is all the more true since public opinion and
even medical personnel still view mental disease as something
shameful, as a stigma. In addition, the authorities want
to humiliate the human dignity of political dissenters.
As is well known, the central goal of concentration camps
was not only to punish but also to break the will of the
prisoners, to deprive them of self-esteem and hope. An
analogous situation, although to a less extent, exists in
special mental hospitals. It is extremely difficult to
maintain one's convictions in a humiliated position. It
is hard for a dissident to preserve his courage when he
is incarcerated in the same ward with psychotics and
criminals, when he is treated as insane and must beg
permission to use the bathroom or to smoke.*

---

* It resembles, to some extent, methods of brainwashing
which were used in North Korea on American prisoners of
war.

Therefore, the authorities found that a psychiatric tendency to interpret any deviations from conventional norms as a sympton of disease, is a very convenient thing. However, one should bear in mind that the number of such cases is not so great as some assume. Charges by certain authors (Tarsis, for example) that Soviet mental hospitals are crammed full of mentally normal political dissenters do not correspond to reality.

The abuse of psychiatry for political purposes began to spread after a series of political trials from 1966 to 1968 which aroused protests at home and abroad. Information about the number of cases of involuntary treatment in psychiatric hospitals is beginning to be known in the West through reports of Russian writers (1-16).

Many of these people are mentally normal. Such dissidents as Grigorenko, Yakhimovich, Bukovskii, Plyushch are highly moral, honest, principled people who have not been frightened by threats and persecution; who have openly expressed their convictions. (If nonconformity, inflexibility, and selflessness are signs of mental illness, then we would declare insane the Christian Saints, Savanorola, Giordano Bruno, Rousseau, Tolstoy, Albert Schweitzer, Dr. King, and other revolutionaries, moralists, and reformers.)

The psychiatric conclusions in these cases were based on doubtful evidences. Let me illustrate with the case of General Grigorenko. He was very disturbed by Khrushchev's reports of Stalin's crimes. He began to state his views and as a result was threatened, persecuted, and finally sent to a psychiatric hospital. The psychiatrist wrote "Grigorenko was always highly principled, energetic, industrious, asserted his views, defended the weak and at the same time overestimated his knowledge and ability, was hot tempered, and always passionately expressed his point of view." This "point of view" demonstrated to the experts his predisposition to psychiatric illness.*

The experts characterized the beginning of the disease as follows: "He thought a great deal about the matters of

---

* Act No. 58/e, Forensic Psychiatric Expertise. See Grigorenko (9), Thoughts of a Madman, pp. 284-294.

the 20th Party Congress and came to the conclusion that all
the followers of the 'cult of personality' had not yet been
totally liquidated. Later he decided that 'the government
is rotting,' having departed from Leninist norms and
principles. He began to express this openly in public
(a sure sign of paranoia to Soviet experts). He was absorbed
by these thoughts and considered this a matter of conscience
and honor."

In conclusion the forensic psychiatrists of the Serbskii
Institute said that Grigorenko's speeches and leaflets
evinced various reformist ideas. In particular his ideas
about reorganizing the Soviet state were evidence of
"paranoia."

Having been adjudged "irresponsible," he was sent for
involuntary treatment in a special psychiatric hospital in
Leningrad. Grigorenko remained there until 1965. After
his discharge he was deprived of his rank and pension since
in the opinion of the KGB and others at the Serbskii Institute he had conducted himself "improperly."   The 60-year-
old general could only find work as a laborer.   He considered that he was suffering for his ideas and continued to
work as a laborer. The experts, of course, considered all
of this absurd. He again began to occupy himself with
socio-political questions, struggled with injustice and
lawlessness and wrote letters to government leaders and
the KGB in which he set forth his point of view. He came
out against the political trials, the occupation of
Czechoslovakia, and defended the rights of the Crimean
Tatars exiled from the Crimea by Stalin.

In 1969 he was sent by the KGB to a forensic
psychiatric commission in Tashkent where he had met with
Crimean Tatars. The commission judged his state of
mental health to be normal (Professor F. F. Detengof).

However,this did not satisfy the KGB and the examination was repeated in the Serbskii Institute in 1969. The
psychiatrists present were G. Morosov, V. Morosov, Lunz,
and others. They indicated that Grigorenko "considered his
struggle completely lawful.... He declared to the doctor
that he cannot abandon his ideas...He formally declared that
he does not number himself among outstanding people." The
experts very much would have liked to expose his "grandiose

ideas." However, they considered that his letters revealed
an evident overestimation of the importance of his
activities. This provided sufficient evidence to reach the
following conclusion: "Grigorenko is suffering from a
psychiatric illness in the form of a pathological
(paranoiac) personality development accompanied by ideas
of reformism, psychopathic peculiarities, and the initial
signs of arteriosclerosis of the vessels of the brain."
Again he was sent for involuntary treatment and he remained
five years, despite his poor physical condition. He was
released at the end of July, 1974, before President Nixon's
arrival in the USSR.

The next example deals with a simple man, unknown in
the West. In Rome I examined an emigrant - K. This young
man had studied in an institute in Leningrad. He had never
seen a psychiatrist. He applied to emigrate to Israel and
was denied permission. He began to take part in the protest
movement and wrote a letter to the government.

Not long before Nixon's visit to Leningrad in 1970, he
was summoned to the military commissariat for psychiatric
examination. When he arrived, he was taken to a separate
room where two men in staff uniforms informed him that he
must undergo an examination in the hospital. He was
detained in a psychiatric hospital for two months despite
his protests. His mother was told in secret by the doctor in
the district psychiatric dispensary that the dispensary
forms which bore the seal and signature of the chief doctor
and by which people were committed to psychiatric
hospitals were obtained from the district KGB.

After his release from the hospital, he received
permission to emigrate. I discovered no symptoms of
mental illness when I examined him. However, he did
manifest certain distinctive personality traits and a
"non-standard style of life," as Adler would say. I cannot
exclude the possibility that information about "peculiarities" received by the KBG and doctors from K.'s colleagues
and other informers served as additional reasons (of
course not the main one) for K.'s incarceration in a
mental hospital.

With such an extremely sensitive attitude toward
political dissidents, forensic psychiatrists find

personality anomalies among many dissidents according to
the Biblical maxim: "Seek and ye shall find." The only
difference is in the diagnosis. If a person was energetic,
active, sociable, but obstinate and rigid, then he was
diagnosed as a paranoiac personality. If the person in
question was independent, somewhat introverted, reserved,
eccentric, his case was diagnosed as schizophrenia (in
various forms). In the latter cases, psychiatrists were
assisted in their diagnosis by the collection of supporting
information about the patient's "strange character," his
"cold" relationship with those nearest to him, his
"inadequate" emotional reactions, special emotional states,
and other vague signs, supposedly indications of
schizophrenia, but in reality characteristic of many people.
The signs of "deranged thought" were no less questionable.
Thus the diagnoses of Yakhimovich, the poet Gorbanevskaya,
the mathematician Plyushch, and others were based on their
"arguments," that is, they ran counter to the special
criteria which psychiatrists proposed for "normal" thought.
The psychiatrist considers himself to be normal and
considers discussions about the terrible fate of people in
labor camps and the need for democratic freedom to be
"futile."

The term "uncritical" was often used in relation to
Yakhimovich, Grigorenko, Borisov, and others. This meant
that the political statements of the accused persons were
considered by the experts to be preposterous: the fact
that the ideas of the accused did not coincide with those
of the experts qualified them as "lacking critical
faculties."

In the case of Borisov, it was stated that he had
"stated his anti-government views harshly,...but was not able
to formulate his own positive program" (as if many people,
even very intelligent ones, were able to formulate their own
political programs). Zhores Medvedev, who has subsequently
emigrated to the West, was released from a psychiatric
hospital only after long and persistent pressure from
Soviet and foreign scientists and writers. Psychiatric
experts had noted that the quality of his work in the field
of genetics had deteriorated in preceding years (as if a
psychiatrist were capable of making such a judgment) and
that in occupying himself with political questions instead
of biology, Medvedev was showing signs of schizophrenia.

However, it is possible to draw another conclusion from the examples presented above: during the examination many psychiatrists are guided by their understanding of medical duty. Thus, for instance, the first examination of General Grigorenko in Tashkent reached a negative conclusion and did not designate him as mentally ill. Therefore it was necessary to direct Grigorenko to the Serbskii Institute of Forensic Psychiatry. For those experts occupying high posts in the Soviet psychiatric hierarchy, the dissident Grigorenko and his active struggle were already signs of paranoid syndrome (although it is hard to say how sincere they were in their judgment).

In the case of K., which I discussed above, the important point turned out to be the fact that the young man had stopped studying, had begun to dress as a "hippy," had grown a beard, etc. To many psychiatrists this is very suspicious in the sense that it marks the beginning of the simple form of schizophrenia. Observing a patient in a psychiatric hospital could not thus contradict their medical conscience.

To ordinary people, among them some doctors and KGB officials, it is a very convincing argument that "thought-less" activities against the gigantic and powerful apparatus of the government which are "lacking in perspective" are indications of mental illness. Since these activities are "crazy," some experts have devised indicators on which to base diagnoses of mental illness. These include "suspicious" symptoms such as beards, eccentric clothes, casual sexual relationships, and other anomalies typical of Bohemian surroundings and modern urban youth.

A psychiatric expert has to be a loyal subject of the state. Thought and behavior in the USSR must be standard; it must conform; it must correspond to the stereotypes of official ideology and customs. Therefore all doubts as to the state's absolute benevolence and the perfection of ideology and government indicate insanity. A priori, a psychiatrist who accepts official ideals must testify to the insanity of political dissidents. In the case against Yakhimovich, the experts denounced the accused, saying that he was struggling against "pseudo-injustice" and that he criticized "pseudo-deficiencies in the government."

Of course, among the dissidents there are many people who deviate from the conventional norm in some ways. But such deviations are typical of many nonconformists and dissenting intellectuals in any country.

Finally, among the dissenters there were also people who were mentally ill. However, it was not necessary to isolate them and they would not have been sent for compulsory treatment if their statements did not have an anti-governmental character.

I would like to emphasize again that not all Soviet psychiatrists are government agents unworthy of the title "doctor." Despite the specific cases described above, the average Soviet psychiatrist is little distinguished from his foreign colleagues in moral and professional levels. As in other countries, in the USSR most doctors owe their first responsibility to the patient. The great bulk of psychiatrists are not involved in involuntary incarceration of dissidents. And some of those who do take part in such activities find "suspicious symptoms" in dissidents and believe that they are serving their medical and patriotic duty (as a result of "internal censorship"). Only in rare cases can one speak of a conscious violation of medical ethics, but even this is socially determined. Although these people deserve thorough condemnation, American public opinion knows that Soviet bureaucrats are not alone in their disregard of moral principles for the sake of a particular group or of private interests.

The abuse of psychiatry reflects an impatience with and a distrust in man. This is typical of a totalitarian regime. Although these attitudes are becoming less common in the USSR, they are still found in all spheres of social and political life: in the fear to grant the people civil rights, in the filtering of "essential" information to be disseminated through the mass media, in censorship, in the propagation of an official ideology, in the declaration of a sanctimonious morality in which no one believes, in a didactic approach to education, and so on.

However, it is paradoxical that the practice of the institutionalization of critics testifies to the weakening of the regime and even to its liberalization. These methods which have evoked such a response in the West are

many times milder than those which were used under Stalin
when millions of completely innocent persons were
physically exterminated.

To sum up, it is possible to explain the causes of the
present "prostitution" of psychiatry in the following
manner:

1. There exists in Russia an old tradition of ignoring
    the rights of the mental patient, which leads
    to the possibility of institutionalization
    and treatment without legal protection. This
    stems from the lack of basic human rights in
    the USSR.

2. Soviet psychiatrists employ an overly broad
    interpretation of the concept of mental
    illness, paranoid states, and schizophrenia,
    including in this framework many different
    deviations from a standard of conformity and
    "well adapted behavior."

3. In a totalitarian society, deviations of
    thought and behavior are considered to be
    signs of criminality or insanity. Under
    Stalin such deviations were always considered
    criminal. Today, they are seen as evidence
    of mistaken ideas or of insanity.

4. Some Soviet psychiatrists, especially the
    leaders, are similar to bureaucrats. The
    bureaucrat is accustomed to respecting
    power and to carrying out all orders of
    authorities. He assumes that he is
    fulfilling his duty.

5. Forced hospitalization is a method
    of discrediting and humiliating political
    dissidents which is convenient for author-
    ities when they want to avoid political
    trials.

It is difficult to say how events will develop. It is
to be hoped that Western pressure and internal social
changes will eventually persuade the regime to curtail its
practice of forced hospitalization of its opponents.

This assumption is supported by the gradual development of pragmatism in Soviet society in recent years, by the reduction of control by the authorities over science, and finally by some adherence to legality.

SUMMARY

The abuse of psychiatry in the Soviet Union is a consequence of the use of psychiatry as a method to protect the state. Although the majority of Soviet psychiatrists do not take part in this shameful practice, the involuntary institutionalization of dissidents as well as of other patients displaying "anti-social behavior" does in fact take place.

In an effort to avoid political trials, the government has attempted to transfer to psychiatrists the burden of stabilizing political life and of struggling with the opposition.

However, this is also facilitated by the acceptance by Russian psychistrists of broad concepts of "mental illness," particularly "paranoiac syndrome" and "schizophrenia." Thus, many nonconformists can be treated as mentally ill.

Furthermore, one must bear in mind the insufficient adherence to legal limitations on involuntary hospitalization in general. The process of eliminating the abuse of psychiatry depends on the democratization of Soviet society and on diminishing governmental control over Soviet psychiatry.

BIBLIOGRAPHY

1. Medvedev, Zh. A Question of Madness. MacMillan, London, 1971

2. Medvedev, R. A. On Compulsory Psychiatric Hospitalization for Political Reasons, Proceedings of the Moscow Human Rights Committee, The International League for the Rights of Man. New York, 1972, pp. 125-133

3. Vol'pin, A. S. An Opinion on R. A. Medvedev's Report, Ibid., pp. 134-179

4. Chalidze, V. N. On the Rights of Persons Declared Mentally Ill, Ibid., pp. 180-218.

5. Feinberg, V. The Letter from the Leningrad "Special" Mental Hospital, Samizdat, Moscow, 1971.

6. Gershuny, V. The Letter from the "Special" Mental Hospital, Samizdat, Moscow, 1971.

7. Medvedev Replies to Prof. J. Ziman, Nature, Vol. 244, Aug. 24, 1974.

8. The Chronicle of Human Rights in the USSR, Khronika Press, Nos. 11, 13, 14, 15, New York.

9. Grigorenko, P. G. Thoughts of a Madman, Herzen Foundation, Amsterdam, 1973.

10. Executions by Madness, Possev-Verlag, Frankfurt/Main, 1971.

11. Voikhanskaya, M., A Psychiatrist's Notebook, No. 1, Sept. 10, 1975, Radio Liberty Special Report, RL 379/75.

12. Khodorovich, T. S., Yu. Orlov. They are Turning L. Plyushch into a Lunatic. Why?, Samizdat, Moscow, March, 1975 (Russkaya Mysl', May 15, 1975).

13. Khodorovich, T. The Escalation of Desperation, Russkaya Mysl', June 5, 1975.

14. Zhitnikova, T. Appeals to the American Astronauts, Russkaya Mysl', July 24, 1975.

15. Khodorovich, T. The Case History of Leonid Plyushch, C. Hurst & Co., London, 1975.

16. Plyushch, Leonid. Excerpts from Statement by Dissident on His Detention in Soviet Mental Hospital, The New York Times, Feb. 4, 1976.

17. Merskey, H. Abuse of Psychiatry, The Times, London, Dec. 12, 1973.

18. Wilby, Peter. Psychiatrists Urged: Boycott Russian
     Meeting, The Observer, London, Sept. 9, 1973.

19. Who is Politically Mad?, The Guardian, London,
     Sept. 8, 1973.

20. Abuse of Psychiatry, British Medical Journal,
     London, Sept. 7, 1973.

21. Sinister Twist in Soviet Psychiatry, The Guardian,
     London, Nov. 11, 1973.

22. Senate Rebuked by Soviet Union over Dissidents, The
     Times, Sept. 8, 1973.

23. Marks, L. Bid to Outlaw Political Abuse of
     Psychiatry, The Observer, May 5, 1974.

24. Reddaway, P. Sakharov. Call to Save Scientist in
     Detention, The Times, Aug. 23, 1974.

25. U. S. Psychiatrists Challenge Russia on Sakharov
     Charges, The Herald Tribune, Sept. 12, 1973.

26. Psychiatry in the Soviet Union, Letters, British
     Medical Journal, July 27, 1974, Aug. 10, 1974.

27. Doctor Decries Psychiatric Jails, The New York
     Times, March 31, 1974.

28. Soviet Approached Therapists, The Washington Post,
     July 12, 1974.

29. Soviet Physicist Pleads for Life of Imprisoned
     Colleague, Psychiatric News, March 20, 1974.

30. Nekrasov, Victor. The Letter to Prof. Snezhnevsky,
     The Sunday Times, March 16, 1975.

31. Cruel Treatment, British Medical Journal, Aug. 9, 1975.

32. Chodoff, P. Involuntary Hospitalization of Political
     Dissenters in the Soviet Union, Psychiatric Opinion,
     Vol. II, No. 1, 1974, pp. 5-19.

33. Declaration of Initiating Committee Against Abuses of
    Psychiatry for Political Purposes, Amnesty Inter-
    national, Symposium on Medical Ethics and Abuses of
    Psychiatry for Political Purposes, Geneva, April, 1975.

34. Kirk, Irina. Interview with Boris Segal, Profiles
    in Russian Resistance, Quadrangle, New York, 1975,
    pp. 130-147.

35. Lopez-Ibor, J. J. The Statement, Psychiatric
    Opinion, Vol. II, No. 1, 1974, p. 35.

36. Tarsis, V. Ya. Testimony, Executions by Madness,
    Possev-Verlag, Frankfurt/Main, 1971, pp. 234-249.

CONTRIBUTORS AND PARTICIPANTS

Josef Brožek, Ph.D., Research Professor of Psychology,
    Lehigh University, Bethlehem, Pennsylvania. Dr.
    Brozek has been actively following and reviewing
    Soviet literature on psychology in the USSR over
    several decades. He is Co-Editor of Psychology in
    the USSR: An Historical Perspective (1972).

Samuel A. Corson, Ph.D., Professor of Psychiatry and Bio-
    physics, Director of the Laboratory of Cerebrovisceral
    Physiology, Department of Psychiatry, The Ohio State
    University, Columbus, Ohio, and a member of the facul-
    ty of the Ohio State University Center for Slavic and
    East European Studies. Dr. Corson has published over
    100 papers in the area of psychobiologic and psycho-
    pharmacologic individuality, neuroendocrine and behav-
    ioral response patterns to avoidable and unavoidable
    psychosocial stressors, modification of violent and
    hyperkinetic behavior, and pet-facilitated psychother-
    apy in a hospital setting and in nursing homes. He is
    Editor of an International Series of Monographs on
    Cerebrovisceral and Behavioral Physiology and Condi-
    tional Reflexes (Pergamon Press) and was Editor-in-
    Chief of the International Journal of Psychobiology,
    1970-73. In 1958 he was a member of a medical-scien-
    tific-cultural exchange mission to the USSR under the
    auspices of the American Friends Service Committee and
    the Friends Medical Society. He has been conducting
    study tours on "Psychiatry and Psychology in the USSR,"
    which included conferences at some of the most presti-
    gious institutes and laboratories in the area of higher
    nervous functions, psychology, and psychiatry in the
    USSR. Dr. Corson was scientific and translation editor·
    of four significant Russian monographs, including the
    volume on Biology and Neurophysiology of the Condi-
    tioned Reflex and its Role in Adaptive Behavior by the
    distinguished Soviet neurophysiologist, Academician
    Peter K. Anokhin.

Elizabeth O'Leary Corson, M.S., Research Associate, Department of Psychiatry, The Ohio State University,
Columbus. Her research interests are in the areas
of psychophysiology and psychopharmacology as related
to psychosocial stress, and in the utilization of pet
animals in resocialization processes.

W. Horsley Gantt, M.D., Associate Professor Emeritus of
Psychiatry, Johns Hopkins University School of Medicine; Professor of Clinical Psychiatry, University
of Maryland School of Medicine; and Senior Scientist,
Pavlovian Research Laboratory, Veterans Administration
Hospital, Perry Point, Maryland. Dr. Gantt is a
pioneer in the development of Pavlovian conditioning
methods in relation to psychiatry in the USA. In
1922-23 Dr. Gantt was Medical Chief of the Leningrad
Unit of the American Relief Administration. There
he became acquainted with I. P. Pavlov and decided
to return to Leningrad in 1924 to work with Pavlov at
the Research Institute of Experimental Medicine where
he remained until 1929. Dr. Gantt was the founder and
Director of the Pavlovian Laboratory at Johns Hopkins
University from 1930 to 1958 and the founder and first
President of the Pavlovian Society of North America.
He is the author of several hundred publications and
several books and the Editor of the Pavlovian Journal
of Biological Science, Soviet Neurology and Psychiatry,
and American Lectures in Objective Psychiatry Series.
Dr. Gantt is one of three living students of Pavlov;
the others are E. A. Asratian, Director of the Insti-
tute of Higher Nervous Activity and Neurophysiology in
Moscow, and E. M. Kreps, Director of the Laboratory of
Comparative Physiology and Biochemistry of the I. P.
Pavlov Institute of Physiology in Leningrad.

Elkhonon Goldberg, Ph.D., Research Fellow, Department of
Neuroscience and the R. F. Kennedy Center for Research
in Mental Retardation and Human Development, Albert
Einstein College of Medicine, Bronx, New York. Dr.
Goldberg completed his doctorate at Moscow University
in 1973 with Professor A. R. Luria, one of the most
distinguished Soviet neuropsychologists. Dr. Goldberg
was editor of Dr. Luria's book, Neuropsychology of
Memory, published in the USSR in 1974.

Ian Gregory, M.D., Professor and Chairman, Department of
    Psychiatry, The Ohio State University College of Med-
    icine, Columbus, Ohio. Dr. Gregory is the author of
    three books and over 30 publications. He is a Fellow
    of the American Psychiatric Association, the Royal
    College of Psychiatrists (Canada), and the Royal
    College of Physicians (Canada).

Jimmie Holland, M.D., Associate Clinical Professor and
    Associate Attending Physician, Department of Psychia-
    try, Montefiore Hospital, Albert Einstein School of
    Medicine, Bronx, New York. Dr. Holland is consultant
    for the National Institute of Alcohol Abuse and Alco-
    holism and the National Institute of Mental Health
    Psychiatry Education Branch. In 1972-73 she worked
    at a psychiatric hospital in Moscow as a consultant
    for the NIMH.

Robert M. Krauss, Ph.D., Professor of Psychology, Columbia
    University, New York, New York. Dr. Krauss was for-
    merly Resident Psychologist at the Bell Telephone
    Laboratories. He is Editor of Experimental Social
    Psychology and author of the introduction and editor
    of a volume of translated articles dealing with social
    psychology in the Soviet Union which appeared as Vol.
    11 (1972-73) of Soviet Psychology and Psychiatry.

Samuel H. Osipow, Professor and Chairman, Department of
    Psychology, The Ohio State University, Columbus, Ohio.
    Dr. Osipow's research interests are in the fields of
    vocational behavior, counseling psychology, and cog-
    nitive functions.

Boris Segal, M.D., Ph.D., Research Fellow, Russian Research
    Center, Harvard University, Cambridge, Massachusetts.
    Dr. Segal was formerly Director of the Department of
    Clinical Psychology and Psychotherapy at the Moscow
    Institute of Psychiatry and Director of the Department
    of Mental Hygiene and Psychotherapy of the Moscow Cen-
    tral Institute of Physical Culture. He is the author
    of over 90 publications and several monographs, chiefly
    in the areas of alcoholism, psychosomatic medicine,
    and the role of personality in psychiatric disorders.

Leon I. Twarog, Ph.D., Professor of Slavic Languages and
     Literatures and Director, Center for Slavic and East
     European Studies, The Ohio State University, Columbus.
     Dr. Twarog was the organizer and first Chairman of the
     Department of Slavic Languages and Literatures at the
     Ohio State University. As Associate Dean of Faculties
     for International Programs he organized the Office of
     International Programs. Under his leadership, the
     Slavic and East European library collection grew from
     3,000 to 160,000 volumes.

Robert H. Wozniak, Ph.D., Assistant Professor, Institute of
     Child Development, and Principal Investigator, Research,
     Development, and Demonstration Center in Education of
     Handicapped Children, University of Minnesota, Minnea-
     polis, Minnesota. Dr. Wozniak's major research inter-
     ests are in cognitive developmental psychology, with
     particular reference to interaction of language and
     cognitive and motor systems in the activity of chil-
     dren. He has also published extensively on comparative
     developments in this area in the USSR and in the West.

Isidore Ziferstein, M.D., Associate Clinical Professor of
     Psychiatry, University of California at Los Angeles;
     member of the faculty of the Southern California
     Psychoanalytic Institute and the Training Institute
     of the Los Angeles Group Psychotherapy Society; and
     Research Consultant at the Postgraduate Center for
     Mental Health, New York. Dr. Ziferstein is a Life
     Fellow of the American Psychiatric Association. His
     major research interests are in group psychotherapy,
     group dynamics, and transcultural psychiatry and he
     has over 50 publications in these areas. In 1963-64
     Dr. Ziferstein spent 13 months in the USSR working at
     the Bekhterev Psychoneurological Research Institute
     in Leningrad as a Fellow of the Foundations Fund for
     Research in Psychiatry.

INDEX

Academic medicine in USSR, 134

Adrenocortical Hormone metabolism, genetics of, 44

Alcohol, per capita consumption of, 183, 184

Alcoholism
addiction phase, 196
adolescents and, 212-214
age groups and, 190, 212-214
alienation and, 211
antabuse therapy and, 198, 241
attitudes of Irish and Russians, 207
boredom and, 214
Church and, 182
conditional reflex therapy and, 198
crime and, 185, 186, 204
criteria and diagnosis of, 195, 196
cultural differences and, 215, 216
diagnostic criteria in the USSR and USA, 235, 236
dictatorship and, 225
disease and, 204, 205
early drinking experience and, 233
epidemiologic study of, 188, 189
ethnic characteristics of, 218-224

Alcoholism (cont'd)
ethnic groups and, 205-207
etiology of, 193-195
family disruption and, 204
group therapy in the USSR and, 237
heredity and, 234, 235
historical factors and, 217, 218
in adolescents and permissiveness, 213
in different Soviet Republics, 189, 190, 192
in Italy and France, 215, 216
in rural population, 182, 183
in the USSR, 181, 187, 188
in urban population, 182
in USSR and USA, 201-215
infrequency in Jews, 233
labor productivity and, 186
Marxism and, 211
medical care and, 198
mental disorders and, 205
methods of prevention, 197-200
Mongolian invasion and, 217, 218
peasant characteristcs and, 218-221
psychoanalysis and, 232, 233
research in USSR and USA, 200, 201
sex and, 190, 214, 215

C2